Head and Neck Ultrasound

Guest Editors

JOSEPH C. SNIEZEK, MD, LTC, MC, USA
ROBERT A. SOFFERMAN, MD

OTOLARYNGOLOGIC CLINICS OF NORTH AMERICA

www.oto.theclinics.com

December 2010 • Volume 43 • Number 6

SAUNDERS an imprint of ELSEVIER, Inc.

W.B. SAUNDERS COMPANY

A Division of Elsevier Inc.

1600 John F. Kennedy Boulevard • Suite 1800 • Philadelphia, Pennsylvania 19103-2899

http://www.theclinics.com

OTOLARYNGOLOGIC CLINICS OF NORTH AMERICA Volume 43, Number 6
December 2010 ISSN 0030-6665, ISBN-13: 978-1-4377-1851-5

Editor: Joanne Husovski
Developmental Editor: Donald Mumford

Otolaryngologic Clinics of North America (ISSN 0030-6665) is published bimonthly by Elsevier, Inc., 360 Park Avenue South, New York, NY 10010-1710. Months of issue are February, April, June, August, October, and December. Business and Editorial Offices: 1600 John F. Kennedy Blvd., Suite 1800, Philadelphia, PA 19103-2899. Customer Service Office: 6277 Sea Harbor Drive, Orlando, FL 32887-4800. Periodicals postage paid at New York, NY and additional mailing offices. Subscription prices is $310.00 per year (US individuals), $590.00 per year (US institutions), $149.00 per year (US student/resident), $409.00 per year (Canadian individuals), $741.00 per year (Canadian institutions), $459.00 per year (international individuals), $741.00 per year (international institutions), $230.00 per year (international & Canadian student/resident). Foreign air speed delivery is included in all *Clinics'* subscription prices. All prices are subject to change without notice. **POSTMASTER:** Send address changes to *Otolaryngologic Clinics of North America*, Elsevier Health Sciences Division, Subscription Customer Service, 3251 Riverport Lane, Maryland Heights, MO 63043. **Telephone: 1-800-654-2452 (U.S. and Canada); 314-447-8871 (outside U.S. and Canada). Fax: 314-447-8029. E-mail: journalscustomerservice-usa@elsevier.com (for print support); journalsonlinesupport-usa@elsevier.com (for online support).**

Reprints. For copies of 100 or more of articles in this publication, please contact the Commercial Reprints Department, Elsevier Inc., 360 Park Avenue South, New York, NY 10010-1710. Tel.: 212-633-3812; Fax: 212-462-1935; E-mail: reprints@elsevier.com.

Otolaryngologic Clinics of North America is also published in Spanish by McGraw-Hill Interamericana Editores S.A., P.O. Box 5-237, 06500 Mexico D.F., Mexico.

Otolaryngologic Clinics of North America is covered in *MEDLINE/PubMed (Index Medicus)*, *Current Contents/Clinical Medicine, Excerpta Medica, BIOSIS, Science Citation Index*, and *ISI/BIOMED*.

Printed and bound by CPI Group (UK) Ltd, Croydon, CR0 4YY

Transferred to Digital Print 2011

Contributors

GUEST EDITORS

JOSEPH C. SNIEZEK, MD, FACS, LTC, MC
USA, Chair, Otolaryngology—Head and Neck Surgery, Tripler Army Medical Center, MCHK-DSH, Honolulu; Associate Clinical Professor, Department of Surgery, John A. Burns School of Medicine, University of Hawaii, Honolulu, Hawaii

ROBERT A. SOFFERMAN, MD, FACS
Professor of Surgery, Division of Otolaryngology, University of Vermont School of Medicine, Fletcher Allen Health Care, Burlington, Vermont

AUTHORS

JEFFREY M. BUMPOUS, MD, FACS
Professor and Chief, Division of Otolaryngology, Department of Surgery, University of Louisville, Louisville, Kentucky

BENJAMIN B. CABLE, MD
Assistant Professor of Surgery, Uniformed Services University of the Health Sciences, Bethesda, Maryland; Pediatric Otolaryngology—Head and Neck Surgery, Tripler Army Medical Center, Honolulu, Hawaii

MARC D. COLTRERA, MD
Professor of Otolaryngology—Head and Neck Surgery, University of Washington Medical Center, Seattle, Washington

MICHAEL R. HOLTEL, MD, FACS
Associate Professor, Telemedicine Research Institute, University of Hawaii; Senior Clinical Advisor, Telemedicine and Advanced Technology Research Center of the United States Army Medical Readiness and Materiel Command Fort Detrick, Maryland

GERALD T. KANGELARIS, MD
Department of Otolaryngology—Head and Neck Surgery, University of California San Francisco, San Francisco, California

THERESA B. KIM, MD
Department of Otolaryngology—Head and Neck Surgery, University of California San Francisco, San Francisco, California; Fellow in Pediatric Otolaryngology, Washington University, St Louis, Missouri

LTC CHRISTOPHER KLEM, MD
Chief, Head and Neck Surgery, Otolaryngology—Head and Neck Surgery Service, Tripler Army Medical Center, Honolulu, Hawaii

LISA LEE, MD
Resident, Department of Otolaryngology—Head and Neck Surgery, University of Cincinnati Medical Center, Medical Sciences Building, Cincinnati, Ohio

LISA A. ORLOFF, MD, FACS
Robert K. Werbe Distinguished Professor in Head and Neck Cancer, Department of Otolaryngology–Head and Neck Surgery, University of California San Francisco, San Francisco, California

GREGORY W. RANDOLPH, MD, FACS
Director, General Otolaryngology Service; Director, Thyroid and Parathyroid Surgical Service, Massachusetts Eye and Ear Infirmary, Boston, Massachusetts

VERONICA J. ROOKS, MD
Assistant Professor of Radiology, Uniformed Services University of the Health Sciences, Bethesda, Maryland; Chief, Pediatric Radiology, Department of Radiology, Tripler Army Medical Center, Honolulu, Hawaii

RUSSELL B. SMITH, MD, FACS
Associate Professor, Department of Otolaryngology–Head and Neck Surgery, University of Nebraska Medical Center; Nebraska Methodist Estabrook Cancer Center, Omaha, Nebraska

JOSEPH C. SNIEZEK, MD, FACS, LTC, MC
USA, Chair, Otolaryngology–Head and Neck Surgery, Tripler Army Medical Center, MCHK-DSH, Honolulu; Associate Clinical Professor, Department of Surgery, John A. Burns School of Medicine, University of Hawaii, Honolulu, Hawaii

ROBERT A. SOFFERMAN, MD, FACS
Professor of Surgery, Division of Otolaryngology, University of Vermont School of Medicine, Fletcher Allen Health Care, Burlington, Vermont

DAVID L. STEWARD, MD
Department of Otolaryngology–Head and Neck Surgery, University of Cincinnati Medical Center, Cincinnati, Ohio

ADVISORS TO OTOLARYNGOLOGIC CLINICS 2010

SAMUEL BECKER, MD
Becker Nose and Sinus Center; Voorhees, New Jersey

DAVID HAYNES, MD
Vanderbilt University; Nashville, Tennessee

BRIAN KAPLAN, MD
Ear, Nose, and Throat Associates; Baltimore, Maryland

JOHN KROUSE, MD, PhD
Temple University Medicine; Philadelphia, Pennsylvania

ANIL KUMAR LALWANI, MD
New York University Langone Medical Center; New York, New York

ARLEN MEYERS, MD, MBA
University of Colorado; Denver, Colorado

MATTHEW RYAN, MD
University of Texas Southwestern Medical Center, Dallas, Texas

RALPH TUFANO, MD
Johns Hopkins Medicine; Baltimore, Maryland

Contents

This article provides an overview of ultrasound and the techniques for its use by otolaryngologists in diagnosing and treating neck masses and lesions. Head and neck ultrasound is extremely useful in diagnosing neck masses and lesions and in facilitating many procedures that are commonly performed on the head and neck. Although in the past these studies were generally performed by radiologists, clinicians are now able to perform high-quality ultrasound studies and ultrasound-guided procedures in the head and neck. Given the advanced knowledge of head and neck anatomy and disease processes that otolaryngologists possess, head and neck ultrasound offers a logical and valuable extension of the physical examination. Recent improvements in ultrasound resolution, portability, and affordability have provided an excellent impetus for otolaryngologists to incorporate ultrasound into their office and operative practices.

This content presents to the neophyte ultrasonographer the essential nutshell of information needed to properly interpret ultrasound images. Basic concepts of physics related to ultrasound are supported with formulas and related to clinical use.

Thorough knowledge of the complex anatomy of the head and neck is essential to understanding the ultrasonographic appearance of this region. The intimate familiarity with anatomic structures obtained by performing surgical procedures makes active radiographic imaging modalities like ultrasound especially suited for use by surgeons. An understanding of the normal sonographic appearance of head and neck structures is critical to recognizing abnormal pathology.

This content is designed to acquaint the clinician with some of the more common ultrasonographic manifestations of clinical conditions that the otolaryngologist is likely to encounter in a general practice. The clinician requires a thorough knowledge of head and neck anatomy to best interpret the variations from normal structures demonstrated on ultrasound. A knowledge of sonographic artifacts may assist the examiner in properly identifying the process under review. Ultrasonography may be the best imaging study for certain organs. In many instances it is the first clinical study that directs further imaging. By providing the clinician with clues as to the underlying pathology, it allows a more efficient direction in determining which aspiration techniques to use.

the clinic and the operating room. Ultrasound offers several advantages to the pediatric patient population. It is well tolerated and adds a degree of precision to the physical examination. It can be done repeatedly as lesions evolve and treatment is performed. It is valuable for guidance and therapeutic treatment of lesions in the operating room. It is likely that ultrasound use will continue to rapidly grow and evolve as a tool within the field of otolaryngology.

Emerging Technology in Head and Neck Ultrasonography   1267

Michael R. Holtel

Increased use of ultrasonography of the head and neck by clinicians has resulted from more compact, higher resolution ultrasound machines that can be more readily used in the office setting. Palm-sized machines are already used for vascular access and bladder assessment. As the resolution of these machines becomes adequate for head and neck assessment, ultrasonography is likely to become a routine adjunct to the office physical examination. Further techniques to reduce artifact beyond spatial compounding, second harmonics, and broadband inversion techniques are likely to be developed to improve ultrasound images. Manual palpation using the ultrasound transducer or "sound palpation," using sound to recreate vibration provides information on tissue "stiffness," which has been successfully used to distinguish between benign and malignant lesions in the head and neck (particularly thyroid nodules). Microbubble contrast-enhanced ultrasound provides improved resolution of ultrasound images. Three- and four-dimensional ultrasonography provides for more accurate diagnosis. The ability of microbubbles with ligands affixed to their outer surface to target specific tissue makes them excellent delivery vehicles. DNA plasmids, chemotherapy agents, and therapeutic drugs can be released at a specific anatomic site. The motion of microbubbles stimulated by ultrasound can be used to increase drug penetration through tissues and has been shown to be effective in breaking up clots in stroke patients (without increased risk). High-intensity focused ultrasound can be used to create coagulation necrosis without significant damage to adjacent tissue. It has been effectively used in neurosurgery and urology, but its effectiveness in the head and neck is still being determined. A prototype for surgical navigation with ultrasound has been developed for the head and neck, which allows real-time imaging of anatomic surgical changes.

THE CLINICS ARE NOW AVAILABLE ONLINE!

Access your subscription at:
www.theclinics.com

Preface

Head and Neck Ultrasound

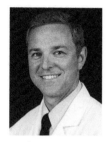 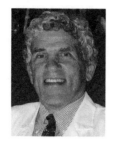

Joseph C. Sniezek, MD   Robert A. Sofferman, MD
Guest Editors

While ultrasound technology continues to emerge as a potent radiologic modality in various aspects of medicine, recent improvements in the clarity (resolution), portability, and cost of ultrasound machines have truly been a game-changer for clinicians who treat maladies of the head and neck. High-quality ultrasound machines are now roughly the size of laptop computers with resolution that approaches the quality of CT scans. Further, the cost of these machines has been reduced to the extent that they are now affordable for most office-based practices. The culmination of these factors has resulted in a condition where ultrasound examinations can and should be performed by clinicians in the setting of both the office and the operating room.

The bottom line is that ultrasound, in the hands of the clinician, allows for a more effective physical examination, improving the accuracy of many diagnoses and often obviating the need for additional tests, studies, and procedures that are frequently more invasive or expensive. Further, clinician-performed ultrasound facilitates and improves many procedures that are commonly performed by the otolaryngologist, such as fine-needle aspiration and abscess drainage. Exciting and novel uses for ultrasound technology are also being explored that promise innovative methods to diagnose and treat neoplasms, infections, and congenital abnormalities of the head and neck.

This volume introduces the otolaryngologist to the basics of head and neck ultrasound, beginning with a primer on the physics of ultrasound. Subsequent articles display the normal anatomy of the head and neck when visualized with contemporary ultrasound as well as the role that ultrasound plays in diagnosing and treating common disorders of the head and neck. Future applications of ultrasound technology are also discussed.

While this volume is by no means exhaustive, it does serve as a testament to the great potential of head and neck ultrasound when placed in the hands of the clinician.

Otolaryngol Clin N Am 43 (2010) ix–x
doi:10.1016/j.otc.2010.09.001
0030-6665/10/$ – see front matter © 2010 Elsevier Inc. All rights reserved.

We hope that it will serve as a reference and inspiration for otolaryngologists who are willing to explore the many advantages of head and neck ultrasound.

Joseph C. Sniezek, MD
Otolaryngology/Head & Neck Surgery
Tripler Army Medical Center, MCHK-DSH
1 Jarrett White Road
Honolulu, HI 96859-5000, USA

Department of Surgery
John A. Burns School of Medicine
University of Hawaii, 651 Ilalo Street
HI 96813, USA

Robert A. Sofferman, MD
Division of Otolaryngology
University of Vermont School of Medicine
Fletcher Allen Health Care
ACC West Pavilion 4th Floor
111 Colchester Avenue
Burlington, Vermont 05401, USA

E-mail addresses:
joseph.sniezek@us.army.mil (J.C. Sniezek)
robert.sofferman@vtmednet.org (R.A. Sofferman)

Head and Neck Ultrasound: Why Now?

Joseph C. Sniezek, MD[a,b,]*

KEYWORDS

• Ultrasound • Head • Neck • Ultrasound-guided procedures

ULTRASOUND IN EVALUATION AND DIAGNOSIS OF NECK MASSES

Although the use and value of ultrasound in the evaluation and diagnosis of neck masses is well accepted by the radiology community, clinicians in the United States have not widely adopted the use of office-based ultrasound in the direct patient care setting of the clinic. European clinicians who treat disorders of the head and neck use office-based ultrasound extensively in outpatient clinics and emergency rooms.

Several roadblocks have precluded ultrasound use by clinicians in the United States. The most profound of these are the perceived steep learning curve, absence of training in head and neck ultrasound in clinical residencies, and perceived scope of practice issues with radiologists. American surgeons only recently have begun to experiment with this technology in the office, because ultrasound was traditionally perceived as difficult to interpret, inaccessible, and the "turf" of specialists in ultrasound radiology. These factors have left American clinicians, both military and civilian, relatively untrained in the use of head and neck ultrasound and totally dependent on the availability of the radiologist to perform ultrasound examinations and ultrasound-guided procedures for head and neck masses and lesions.

Recent improvements in the quality of resolution of ultrasound units has rendered the interpretation of ultrasound images much easier, with results that approach the clarity of CT scanning at a fraction of the cost and time. Head and neck ultrasound training and instructor training courses are also now offered at medical meetings in the United States. The combination of the increased ease of use of contemporary ultrasound units and the availability of surgeon-instructors has finally engendered

---

This work was supported by a grant from the AMEDD Advancements in Medical Technology Initiative (AAMTI).

[a] Otolaryngology/Head & Neck Surgery, Tripler Army Medical Center, MCHK-DSH, 1 Jarrett White Road, Honolulu, HI 96859-5000, USA

[b] Department of Surgery, John A. Burns School of Medicine, University of Hawaii, 651 Ilalo Street, HI 96813, USA

* Corresponding author. Otolaryngology/Head & Neck Surgery, Tripler Army Medical Center, MCHK-DSH, 1 Jarrett White Road, Honolulu, HI 96859-5000.
E-mail address: joseph.sniezek@us.army.mil

Otolaryngol Clin N Am 43 (2010) 1143–1147
doi:10.1016/j.otc.2010.08.001
0030-6665/10/$ – see front matter. Published by Elsevier Inc.

guarded interest among clinicians. Of similar importance, the cost of portable ultrasound machines with excellent resolution and straightforward functionality has recently decreased, making them now affordable for most office practices.

Given the recent improvements in ultrasound resolution and the affordability of portable ultrasound units, clinician-performed head and neck ultrasound now offers otolaryngologists the opportunity to improve the quality and efficiency of patient care in several ways. This article introduces some of these methods, with much more in-depth discussions provided in other articles elsewhere in this issue.

OFFICE-BASED ULTRASOUND

Contemporary portable ultrasound units have become smaller, much easier to interpret, and less expensive, with many models costing less than $30,000. This improved accessibility of ultrasound technology has enabled clinicians to finally have a tool that improves the physical examination of patients, literally enabling clinicians to see what lies beneath the skin during an initial patient evaluation. Clinicians are now able to accurately risk-stratify thyroid nodules based on their appearance on ultrasound, complementing the information obtained on fine needle aspiration biopsies.[1–5] Furthermore, subcutaneous masses, such as adenopathy or abscesses, can be accurately diagnosed, followed up, or treated, helping otolaryngologists to quickly and inexpensively formulate the most appropriate management course.

In the past, most otolaryngologists would immediately order a CT, MRI, or radiologist-performed ultrasound scan on diagnosing a neck mass. This prescription would often require patients to wait days to weeks for the imaging to be scheduled, performed, and interpreted before they could return to the office for a follow-up appointment to discuss the disease process. Now, an ultrasound can be immediately performed by otolaryngologists during the initial visit, allaying patient anxiety and obviating any delays in treatment.

ULTRASOUND-GUIDED PROCEDURES

Ultrasound is extremely useful in facilitating various procedures in the head and neck that otolaryngologists commonly perform (**Fig. 1**). Ultrasound guidance has been shown to increase the sensitivity and specificity of fine needle aspiration (FNA) biopsies of head and neck lesions compared wit traditional palpation-guided techniques, particularly in the thyroid and parotid glands.[6–8] Although much of the literature addresses ultrasound guidance performed by a radiologist, contemporary studies indicate that in the hands of an otolaryngologist, a similar improvement in FNA technique and results occurs when ultrasound guidance is used.[9] Similarly, ultrasound helps guide needle placement during core needle biopsies, improving the diagnostic accuracy and safety of the procedure.

Ultrasound may also improve the diagnosis and treatment of head and neck infections and abscesses.[10] Liquefactive necrosis is fairly easily identified on ultrasound, aiding in the diagnosis of an abscess. Ultrasound can also help guide the needle during needle aspiration of abscesses, and help identify when an adequate drainage has occurred.[11] This technique is particularly helpful in draining pediatric abscesses, given the small size and proximity to vital structures. Minor abscess drainage may even be performed in the clinic or intensive care unit setting, occasionally eliminating the need for a trip to the operating room.

One novel use of head and neck ultrasound is in the minimally invasive treatment of head and neck vascular lesions. Under ultrasound guidance, a flexible laser probe can be inserted through an angiocatheter, selectively targeting vascular lesions in the head

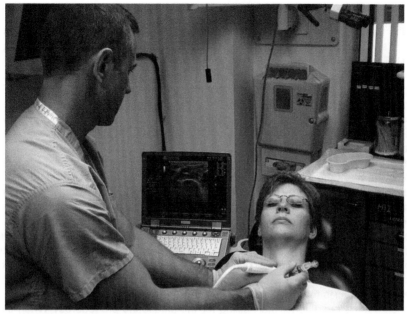

Fig. 1. Portable ultrasound units greatly facilitate office-based procedures, such as ultrasound-guided fine needle aspiration biopsy.

and neck. This technique is highlighted in the article by Dr Cable on Pediatric Applications of Head and Neck Ultrasound found elsewhere in this issue.

ULTRASOUND IN MILITARY/RURAL SETTINGS

In the military, in particular, ultrasound has become incredibly appealing. As ultrasound technology has improved in clarity and resolution, it has also become packaged in highly portable and durable units, some no larger than a laptop computer. This enhanced quality and improved portability has led to the placement of an ultrasound unit in every Army Forward Surgical Team and Combat Support Hospital. Likewise, otolaryngologist-performed ultrasound is extremely helpful in rural settings where radiologists are not readily available to perform the procedures, particularly in emergency situations.

ULTRASOUND USE IN OPERATIVE PROCEDURES

Beyond the outpatient or clinic setting, ultrasound is also efficacious in various operative procedures. The most well-documented use of head and neck ultrasound in the perioperative setting may be in the identification and localization of parathyroid adenomas. This information is well addressed in the content presented by Dr Steward on Parathyroid Localization elsewhere in this issue. Multiple studies have concluded that ultrasound is superior to CT and sestamibi scans in the preoperative localization of parathyroid adenomas.[12] Furthermore, ultrasound can be extremely helpful in the operative setting, aiding incision placement and intraoperative localization of difficult parathyroid lesions.

GETTING STARTED WITH HEAD AND NECK ULTRASOUND

Adding head and neck ultrasound to one's practice usually begins with attending a Head and Neck Ultrasound Course sponsored by the American College of Surgeons (ACS). The 1-day courses are offered at every ACS meeting and are now delivered throughout the United States in various venues throughout the year. Exported versions of the ACS Head and Neck Ultrasound Course have been delivered in Hawaii and San Francisco at the American Academy of Otolaryngology-Head and Neck Surgery annual meeting, and in conjunction with Triological Society meetings. The only prerequisite for attending one of the courses is the completion of the CD-based ACS Basic Ultrasound course.

After the Head and Neck Ultrasound Course is completed, the next step is to perform as many head and neck ultrasound procedures as possible, tracking the results and discoveries. At first, confirming ultrasound findings with other imaging studies, such as CT or radiologist-performed ultrasounds, might be a significant confidence booster. Practitioners may also decide to borrow a machine used by a colleague who has already added ultrasound to the practice, such as an endocrinologist or surgeon, before personally investing in an ultrasound unit. Another suggestion is for practitioners to query the experience of physicians in their region who use ultrasound, ascertaining opinions of the service quality and availability offered by the different companies that market ultrasound units in the area.

When does a practitioner start billing for the ultrasound procedures? When ultrasound studies performed affect or determine patient care, the procedures may be coded and billed. All ultrasound studies should be documented and a record preserved, just as with any radiologic or diagnostic procedure. Coding and reimbursement rates for ultrasound studies and ultrasound-guided procedures vary by region, of course, but the improvements in patient care in terms of quality, safety, and convenience are universal.

ULTRASOUND AS A TOOL FOR THE OTOLARYNGOLOGIST

The availability, affordability, and usability of portable ultrasound units have recently undergone dramatic improvements. These advances now offer otolaryngologists a portable tool that increases diagnostic accuracy, facilitates commonly performed procedures, and adds to patient convenience and safety. Given the knowledge of head and neck anatomy that otolaryngologists possess, along with the burgeoning number of head and neck ultrasound training courses, adding ultrasound to an otolaryngology practice has never been easier or made more sense.

REFERENCES

1. Papini E, Gugleilmi R, Bianchini A, et al. Risk of malignancy in nonpalpable thyroid nodules: predictive value of ultrasound and color-Doppler features. J Clin Endocrinol Metab 2002;87(5):1941–6.
2. Popowicz B, Klencki M, Lewinski A, et al. The usefulness of sonographic features in selection of thyroid nodules for biopsy in relation to the nodule's size. Eur J Endocrinol 2009;161(1):103–11.
3. Horvath E, Majlis S, Rossi R, et al. An ultrasonogram reporting system for thyroid nodules stratifying cancer risk for clinical management. J Clin Endocrinol Metab 2009;94(5):1748–51.
4. Alexander EK. Approach to the patient with a cytologically indeterminate thyroid nodule. J Clin Endocrinol Metab 2008;93(11):4175–82.

5. Moon WJ, Jung SL, Lee JH, et al. Benign and malignant thyroid nodules: US differentiation—multicenter retrospective study. Radiology 2008;247(3):762–70.
6. Mehanna HM, Jain A, Morton RP, et al. Investigating the thyroid nodule. BMJ 2009;338:b733.
7. Izquierdo R, Arekat MR, Knudson PE, et al. Comparison of palpation-guided versus ultrasound-guided fine-needle aspiration biopsies of thyroid nodules in an outpatient endocrinology practice. Endocr Pract 2006;12(6):609–14.
8. Morris LF, Ragavendra N, Yeh MW. Evidence-based assessment of the role of ultrasonography in the management of benign thyroid nodules. World J Surg 2008;32(7):1253–63.
9. Robitschek J, Straub M, Wirtz E, et al. Diagnostic efficacy of surgeon-performed ultrasound-guided fine needle aspiration: a randomized controlled trial. Otolaryngol Head Neck Surg 2010;142(3):306–9.
10. Kreutzer EW, Jafek BW, Johnson ML, et al. Ultrasonography in the preoperative evaluation of neck abscesses. Head Neck Surg 2006;4(4):290–5.
11. Yusa H, Yoshida H, Ueno E, et al. Ultrasound-guided surgical drainage of face and neck abscesses. Int J Oral Maxillofac Surg 2002;31(3):327–9.
12. Steward DL, Danielson GP, Afman CE, et al. Parathyroid adenoma localization: surgeon-performed ultrasound versus sestamibi. Laryngoscope 2009;116(8):1380–4.

Ultrasound Physics in a Nutshell

Marc D. Coltrera, MD

KEYWORDS

• Ultrasound • Physics • Sound waves • Doppler • Transducer

An understanding of ultrasound physics is essential for the proper interpretation of ultrasound images. Ultrasonic imaging relies on the reflection of sound occurring at the interface between tissues with different acoustical characteristics. Artifacts are common and can help or hinder diagnosis. To properly interpret the images, the ultrasonographer needs to have an understanding of the underlying sound wave. The intent of this content is to supply the minimum, the nutshell, of information needed to help a neophyte ultrasonographer. On first blush, the formulas may appear intimidating but they are meant to illustrate the physical relationships that affect and inform clinical ultrasound. The casual reader is invited to refer to them sparingly. For those who wish to know more, there are many in-depth analyses of ultrasound physics as applied in the clinical setting and several suggestions for additional reading are listed at the end of this article.

SOUND WAVES

Sound waves are created by the propagation of vibrational energy through gas, liquid, or solid: molecules striking molecules. Measured from a single location, the mass molecular movements are detected as pressure waves alternating between compression and rarefaction as the vibrations pass by (**Fig. 1**). Each repetition of the pressure wave is called a cycle. The two fundamental properties used to describe a wave are its wavelength and frequency.

Wavelength

Wavelength (λ) is the distance between like points on the wave occurring once per cycle. For a stationary observer, the time it takes for a complete wave to pass or a cycle to occur is called the wave's period (T). The most common time scale used for sound waves is expressed in seconds, which means T is expressed in units of seconds per cycle. It is easier to use the inverse of the wave's period, its frequency (f), when comparing waves. For a wave with a period of $T = 0.01$ sec/cycle, $f = 1/T = 1/.01 = 100$ cycles/sec. The combination of cycles per second is further simplified by using

Department of Otolaryngology-Head and Neck Surgery, Box 356515, University of Washington Medical Center, 1959 NE Pacific Street, Seattle, WA 98195, USA
E-mail address: coltrera@u.washington.edu

Otolaryngol Clin N Am 43 (2010) 1149–1159
doi:10.1016/j.otc.2010.08.004
0030-6665/10/$ – see front matter © 2010 Elsevier Inc. All rights reserved.

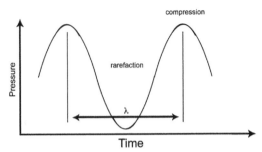

Fig. 1. The sound wave consists of a varying pressure wave passing through a media. The distance between similar points on the curve is the wavelength (λ).

the common unit, the hertz (Hz), where 1 Hz equals 1 cycle/sec. For higher frequencies, kilohertz (kHz = 1000 Hz) and megahertz (MHz = 1,000,000 Hz) are used.

Sonic Range

The audible or sonic range is defined as 20 Hz to 20,000 Hz (20 kHz), the range of human hearing. By convention, frequencies above the range of human hearing are defined as ultrasonic. The most common frequencies used for diagnostic head and neck ultrasound range from 7.5 to 15.0 MHz. The choice of this range is a direct consequence of the physics, as discussed later.

Clinical ultrasonography relies on the measurement of reflected energy. Sound wave reflectance occurs essentially because of alterations in the speed of sound in different media or tissues. Understanding how the speed of sound changes is fundamental to understanding clinical ultrasound.

Propagation Velocity

The speed of a wave is called the propagation velocity. In the case of radiographs, the waves travel at the speed of light, which is 299,792,458 m/sec in a vacuum. Even the speed of light is not constant. It changes in denser materials because of propagating wave conversion into a hybrid of electromagnetic radiation and subatomic particle oscillations. The frequency of the light has effects at the quantum level, which in turn affect the speed of the light wave. Sound waves act at the molecular level. Frequency has no effect on propagation velocity for sound. The two are related by the following simple formula:

$$c = f\lambda$$

where c is the propagation velocity, f is the frequency, and λ is the wavelength.

Two factors that do affect the speed of sound are the (1) density of the medium and (2) elasticity or stiffness of the medium as expressed in the following formula:

$$c = C/\rho$$

where c is the propagation velocity, C is the coefficient of stiffness, and ρ is the density of the medium.

Fig. 2 lists the propagation velocity of typical media encountered in the body. At first glance it might appear confusing that the propagation velocities increase in the denser media because the velocity is inversely proportional to the density (bone velocity > soft tissue velocity > air velocity). The reason is that the stiffness of these media increases

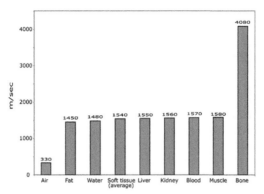

Fig. 2. Sound propagation velocities in air and in typical tissues. The average propagation velocity of 1540 m/sec is a good approximation of most tissue mass in the head and neck region.

much faster than their density does. In general, the speed of sound increases when going from a gas to a liquid to a solid.

Two clinical ultrasound measurements are directly dependent on the speed of propagation:

1. Distance measurement
2. Resolution.

When measuring distance, the time required for sound to return to the transducer multiplied by its speed gives the distance (**Fig. 3**). But, as noted, the speed of sound varies within different tissues based on density and stiffness. Because there is no way for ultrasound designers to know what tissues will be examined, ultrasound machines base distance calculations on an average speed for the expected tissues. The typical

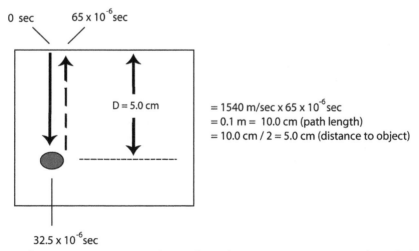

Fig. 3. The average propagation velocity of sound in tissue, 1540 m/sec, is used to calculate distances. A large percentage of fat with a propagation velocity of 1450 m/sec can significantly affect the calculations.

value used is 1540 m/sec, which is derived from averaging fat, liver, kidney, blood, and muscle.[1] This value is a reasonable approximation for the majority of the soft tissues encountered in the neck. In an obese individual with a large percentage of neck fat tissue, actual and measured distances can be significantly different: 1450 (fat propagation velocity)/1540 (average tissue propagation velocity) = 6% differential.

The second clinical measurement depending on the speed of sound is the ability to resolve between two closely spaced points. The ability to distinguish between two points requires a wavelength of the same size or smaller than the distance between the two points (**Fig. 4**). Resolution requirements quickly constrain the choice of frequency of ultrasound for clinical head and neck imaging. Recall the relationship between propagation velocity, frequency, and wavelength:

$$c = f\lambda$$

Using the average propagation speed in the head and neck and plugging in a frequency of 7.5 MHz yields

$$\lambda = c/f = 1540 \text{ m sec}^{-1}/7,500,00 \text{ cycles} \cdot \text{sec}^{-1} = 0.205 \text{ mm}$$

Structures, such as lymph nodes and the parathyroids, are typically in the range of 3 to 4 mm in size. If there were no technical issues to consider, a single cycle of sound energy at 7.5 MHz would be more than adequate for resolving head and neck structures. Unfortunately, single cycle detection is impractical in reality. The transducer material used to create the sound energy acts like a bell. Striking it to start the ringing is simple, but like a bell it is difficult to dampen the induced vibrations after one cycle.

Acoustic Impedance and Reflectance

Clinical ultrasonography equipment relies on reflected sound measurements. Sound wave reflection occurs at the boundary between materials with different acoustic properties. The intrinsic property defining this difference is acoustic impedance (Z), which is the product of the density and the propagation velocity of a medium:

$$Z = \rho c$$

The greater the difference in impedances, the greater the amount of energy that is reflected. Because impedance is a product of density and propagation velocity, the greatest reflectance in the head and neck region is to be expected at air/soft tissue interfaces and bone/soft tissue interfaces. In contrast, ultrasound transducer gels closely match soft tissue impedance, allowing transmission of the sound energy through to the soft tissue with minimal reflectance.

If all reflected energy was returned to the sound detector, all differences between object appearances would be related to their relative impedance. But sound waves

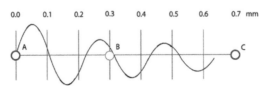

Fig. 4. Axial resolution is theoretically limited by the wavelength of sound energy being employed (*A* → *B*). In practice, the piezoelectric element used to generate the sound energy rings for 2 to 3 cycles and becomes the limiting factor for axial resolution (*A* → *C*).

can be scattered in a manner where they do not return to the detector. Reflectors fall into 2 broad categories:

1. Specular
2. Diffuse.

A specular reflector is one that acts like a mirror. The classic specular reflector is smooth and large compared with the wavelength of the sound wave used to image it. Examples of specular reflectors include the diaphragm, the carotid artery, and fluid-filled cysts. Specular reflectors that are perpendicular to the sound wave's propagation path reflect directly back to the transducer. Angled reflectors will reflect the sound energy away from the transducer leading to a loss of signal (**Fig. 5**).

Diffuse reflectors are common in the head and neck region and account for the speckled patterns seen on ultrasound images. Sound energy is scattered rather than reflected in a coherent manner when the wavelength of the sound wave is larger than the size of the reflector (eg, 0.205 mm for a 7.5 MHz sound wave).

Attenuation

Diagnostic ultrasound imaging relies on the return of sound wave energy to the transducer. In addition to the scattering that occurs with diffuse reflectors and the angled reflectance caused by specular reflectors, another major source of energy loss is attenuation. Absorbance of the sound energy along the path of the wave limits the potential depth of penetration. Tissues absorb sound energy by converting the sound energy into heat. This conversion increases with the frequency of the sound wave and becomes the major factor limiting the depth of tissue penetration when using higher ultrasonic frequencies. As previously discussed, resolution sets a lower limit on the useful range of ultrasound frequencies for the head and neck region. Absorbance, the chief cause of attenuation, sets the upper limit.

Attenuation of the sound wave is measured in relative units based on the intensity levels of sound energy at two points along the propagation path. Intensity is a measure of how power is spread over an area:

$$\text{Power}(\text{in milliwatts } [mW]/\text{Area}(\text{in cm}^2)) = I(\text{Intensity in mW/cm}^2)$$

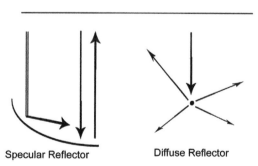

Specular Reflector   Diffuse Reflector

Fig. 5. Smooth acoustic surfaces significantly larger than the ultrasonic wavelengths act as mirrors (specular reflector) reflecting sound energy directly back to the transducer or deflect it. Small acoustic objects smaller than the ultrasonic wavelength scatter the sound energy (diffuse reflector).

The degree of attenuation is expressed in a relative unit, the decibel (dB). The decibel is defined as $10 \times \log_{10}(I_2/I_1)$. If the intensity measured at I_1 is 100 mW/cm^2 and at I_2 is 0.01 mW/cm^2, the attenuation between the two points is

$$10 \times \log_{10}(0.01/100) = 10 \times \log_{10}(0.0001) = -40 \text{ dB}$$

Fig. 6 lists the attenuation values for common media encountered in the body. Air has a high attenuation coefficient because carbon dioxide has a high-absorbance cross section for ultrasonic sound waves. Although soft tissues have much better attenuation values, typical soft tissue attenuation is still enough to significantly limit the penetration depth of higher frequency ultrasound needed to visualize smaller structures. Using an average soft tissue attenuation value of 0.70 dB/cm/MHz, a 7.5 MHz beam at the thyroid's depth of 5 cm results in an attenuation of more than 25 dB. The 12 MHz or higher frequencies needed for visualization of normal parathyroids result in attenuation values greater than 45 dB at the same depth.

The fact that the reflected wave is subject to the same attenuation as it passes back through the overlying tissues doubles tissue attenuation effects. To compensate for the weakened reflections and more closely represent the true characteristics of the deep tissues, differential amplification of signals based on their distance can be employed in an attempt to normalize the signals. Distance calculations are based on the time for the reflected wave to return to the transducer; the differential amplification is referred to as time-gain compensation (TGC;). The limiting factor in TGC is the signal-to-noise ratio, which approaches 1.0 at depths seen in the head and neck with the frequencies in use.

Doppler

In addition to timing the reflected wave, the reflected sound waves contain information encoded in their amplitude, phase, and frequency. B-scale ultrasonography is based on the amplitude of the reflected wave. The greater the amplitude, the brighter the image on the gray scale monitor. Phase changes can be used for motion detection, but the most commonly employed method of motion detection depends on frequency shifts, the Doppler effect (**Fig. 7A**).

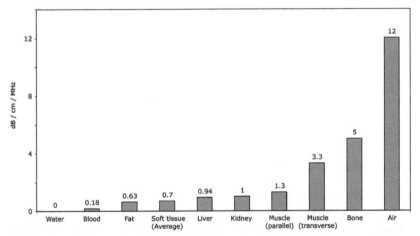

Fig. 6. Attenuation of sound energy within tissues varies with the frequency of the sound. Contributors to attenuation include reflection, scattering, and absorbance.

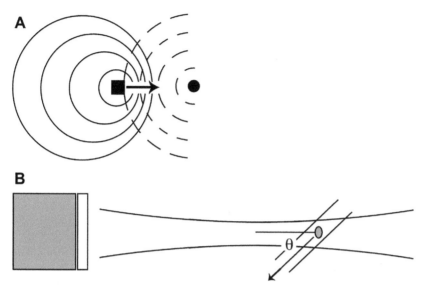

Fig. 7. The Doppler shift is a function of the velocity of the object (*A*) as well as the component of the velocity, which is aligned with the transducer beam (*B*).

The classic example of the Doppler shift is a train whistle that goes from high to low pitch as the train approaches, passes, and then recedes from the observer. The same effect would occur if the observer is moving and the whistle is stationary. If both whistle and observer are moving, the basic Doppler formula includes a factor of 2x to compensate because the frequency shift is effectively doubled.

This factor of 2x is needed to account for the effects seen in clinical ultrasonography. As an observer, the moving blood cell within a blood vessel would experience the classic Doppler shift applied to the incoming ultrasound wave. However, in truth, the blood cell is not the observer. It reflects the Doppler-shifted wave and becomes a moving transmitter that adds a second Doppler shift to the wave when it is finally received by the transducer, which is the true observer. The appropriate Doppler shift formula used in clinical ultrasonography is

$$f_D \approx f_0(2v/(c\text{-}v)) \approx f_0(2v/c)$$

where f_D is Doppler shift, f_0 is source frequency, c is propagation velocity, and v is reflector speed.

Because the typical velocities (v) associated with blood flow are at most a few percent of the average propagation velocity of the ultrasound wave (1540 m/sec [c]), the denominator can be simplified to ($2v/c$).

As a consequence of the Doppler formula, it is apparent that Doppler shift only occurs if the reflector's motion has a component of velocity in the direction of the ultrasound probe (see **Fig. 7**B). The Doppler shift must be corrected for the angle formed between the direction of flow and the ultrasound beam if quantitative velocity analysis of blood is necessary:

$$f_D = f_0(2V/c)\cos\theta$$

In typical head and neck ultrasonography, the most common use of Doppler frequency information is in combination with B-mode ultrasonography. This combination is called color-flow Doppler imaging wherein the stationary B-mode structures are overlaid with a Doppler frequency map. Relative velocity and direction on the Doppler frequency map is conveyed through the use of a color palate ranging from red (flow direction toward the transducer) to blue (flow direction away from the transducer).

Signal-to-noise issues readily affect color-flow Doppler images. Sources of noise include pulsating vessel wall expansion and operator-induced movements. To minimize these problems, signal filtering is employed to exclude low-rate movements. The downside is that low-flow vessels, such as small veins, are excluded in color-flow Doppler images. An alternative to standard Doppler frequency mapping is an integrated power map of the Doppler signal called power-mode Doppler. Although increased signal-to-noise ratios allow for more gain, it comes with the loss of direction and velocity information.

THE PHYSICS OF TRANSDUCER DESIGN

All modern transducers incorporate piezoelectric elements combining the functions of transmitter and receiver for the production and detection of ultrasonic sound waves. These functions do not occur simultaneously, but rather sequentially. The piezoelectric phenomenon was discovered by Pierre Curie in 1880. When placed under mechanical stress, some crystals and ceramic materials generate a voltage. When an external voltage is applied to them they exhibit the reverse phenomenon and undergo a small mechanical deformation (**Fig. 8**). World War I saw the first practical use of the piezoelectric effect in the development of sonar using a separate sound generator and detector. Ultrasonic transducers in clinical applications use the same piezoelectric element to produce the sound energy and then detect the reflected sound waves.

As previously discussed, the ability to resolve two close objects along the propagation path is dependent on the ultrasound frequencies employed. But practical resolution in a 3-dimensional world is greatly dependent on transducer design and its fundamental component, the piezoelectric element. With respect to the transducer beam, the 3 spatial dimensions are: axial, lateral, and elevation (or azimuth) (**Fig. 9**).

Axial resolution is measured along the beam axis and coincides with the propagation path. A 7.5 MHz single-cycle pulse has a 0.205 mm wavelength, but the

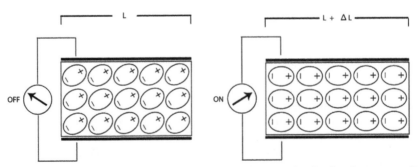

Fig. 8. Application of a voltage to a piezoelectric crystal causes the dipolar elements to align with the applied field alternating the shape of the crystal and leading to a size change ($\triangle$ L). Repeated expansion and contraction of the crystal generates the sound waves. Conversely, reflected sound energy can change the shape of a small crystal inducing a synchronized voltage variation.

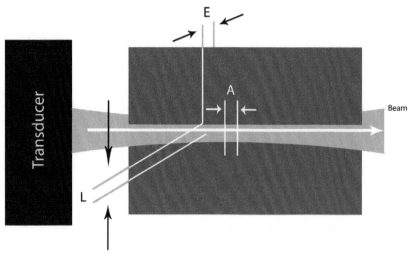

Fig. 9. Beam resolution is measured in 3 planes relative to the transducer orientation: Axial (A), elevation (E, [or azimuth]), and lateral (L). Axial resolution is measured along the beam axis. Lateral resolution is measured in the plane, which is perpendicular to the beam and parallel to the transducer. Elevation resolution, evaluating the thickness of the beam, is measured in the plane perpendicular to both the beam axis and the transducer axis.

piezoelectric element generating the pulse will ring for one or two additional cycles after an applied voltage is discontinued. The complete length of the pulse train determines the achievable axial resolution (see **Fig. 4**). In the case of small objects, such as parathyroids in the range of 2 to 3 mm, a minimum effective resolution of 0.615 mm is not adequate. Although higher frequencies improve resolution, attenuation becomes the limiting factor.

Lateral resolution and elevation resolution are functions of the physical dimensions of the piezoelectric element and as such are typically less than the achievable axial resolution. To a first approximation, lateral resolution is governed by the width of the piezoelectric elements within the transducer. The pressure wave generated by the piezoelectric element's face spreads out with increasing depth further degrading resolution. The depth can be partially compensated for by focusing the ultrasonic beam at the depth of interest through beam timing.

Elevation resolution is dependant on the thickness of the beam measured in the plane perpendicular to the beam axis and the transducer axis. Because the piezoelectric element has edges, the primary pressure wave is generated by the center of the element with less intense side-lobe energy waves given off at the margins. The side lobes can interact with strong reflectors out of the primary beam plane creating artifacts.

Because the transducer is generating the ultrasound pulse and detecting the reflected waves, sufficient time must be allowed for reflected signals to return to the transducer before generating the next pulse. Tissue propagation speed limits the rate that pulses can be generated by the transducer. The rate at which pulses can be created by the transducer is called the pulse repetition frequency (PRF). In the neck, maximal achievable depths caused by attenuation are approximately 7.5 cm, resulting in a total path length of 15 cm and a maximal PRF of 1540 m/sec^{-1}/0.15 m = 10 kHz. Tissue attenuation actually helps increase PRF by minimizing the reflectance of deeper objects.

THE PHYSICS OF ARTIFACTS

Reverberation, multipath, shadowing, enhancement, side lobe, and refraction are the most common artifacts in B-mode ultrasound.

Reverberation artifacts occur when the sound waves repeatedly reflect between two interfaces with significantly mismatched impedances. In the head and neck region, the most commonly encountered reverberation artifact occurs at the tracheal rings (**Fig. 10**). The anterior soft-tissue-to-cartilage interface and the posterior cartilage-to-air interface lead to serial reflections with a resulting artifactual increase in apparent path length.

Multipath artifacts occur at specular reflectors altering the apparent position and shape of objects (see **Fig. 10**). The small specular reflectors in the head and neck region, such as the carotid artery, rarely lead to significant multipath artifacts.

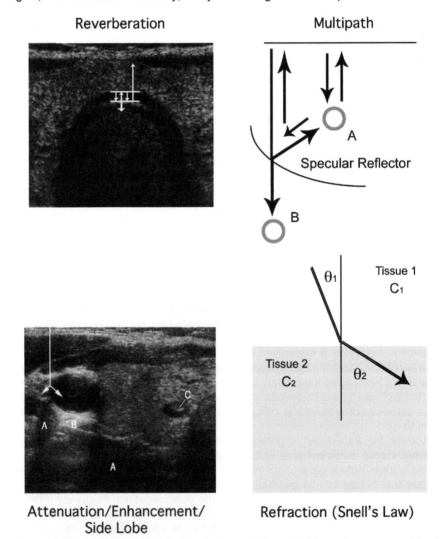

Fig. 10. Common artifacts of B-scale ultrasonography include reverberation, multipath, shadowing (*A*), enhancement (*B*), side lobe (*C*), and refraction.

Shadowing artifacts result from the attenuation of sound energy leading to little or no reflections being returned from deeper objects because of a lack of sound energy. Attenuation can occur through energy absorbance (eg, thick muscles) or through reflectance off an object, such as thyroid calcifications or vessel sidewalls. Conversely, enhancement artifacts occur when the attenuation of overlying tissues is less than surrounding tissues. Fluid-filled cysts and blood within blood vessels have significantly lower attenuation values than surrounding soft tissues leading to enhancement of the deeper tissues (see **Fig. 10**).

Side-lobe artifacts arise when there are strong reflectors just outside the primary beam path. Reflection off a cyst wall outside the sonographic plane can make it appear that there is a mass within the cyst, for example (see **Fig. 10**). Refraction requires the introduction of the last physics formula, Snell's law:

$$\sin\theta_1 / \sin\theta_2 = c_1 / c_2$$

where θ_1 is the angle of incidence approaching the interface, θ_2 is the angle of refraction leaving the interface, c_1 is the propagation velocity in Medium 1, and c_2 is the propagation velocity in medium 2.

The change in direction of propagation occurs when a sound wave passes between two media with different propagation velocities (see **Fig. 10**). Like multipath artifacts, refraction artifacts move the position of objects resulting in spurious duplicates. Significant refraction artifacts are uncommon in the head and neck region, but can be seen at muscle edges.

FURTHER READINGS

Brant William E. The core curriculum: ultrasound. Philadelphia: Lippincott Williams & Wilkins; 2001.

Coltrera MD. In: Lisa Orloff, editor. Essential physics of ultrasound in head and neck ultrasound. San Diego (CA): Plural Publishing; 2008.

Rumack Carol M, Wilson Stephanie R, Charboneau JW, et al, editors. Diagnostic ultrasound. Philadelphia: Elsevier Mosby; 2005.

REFERENCE

1. Chivers RC, Parry RJ. Ultrasonic velocity and attenuation in mammalian tissues. J Acoust Soc Am 1978;63:940–53.

Head and Neck Anatomy and Ultrasound Correlation

Christopher Klem, MD

KEYWORDS
- Ultrasound • Head and neck • Normal anatomy

ULTRASOUND OF HEAD AND NECK: ANATOMY

Ultrasonography of the head and neck has been performed for decades, primarily by radiologists. Recent improvements in high-resolution ultrasound have made the technology much more accessible to clinicians. Office-based ultrasound allows clinicians to personally perform a real-time diagnostic radiographic procedure and literally see pathology below the skin. This ability makes ultrasound an important extension of the physical examination and enables clinicians to more rapidly and effectively treat patients.

A thorough knowledge of the complex anatomy of the head and neck is essential to understanding the ultrasonographic appearance of this region. The frequent performance of surgical procedures leads to a familiarity with anatomic structures that makes active radiographic imaging like ultrasound especially suited for use by surgeons. It is important to understand and appreciate the normal sonographic appearance of head and neck structures before recognizing abnormal pathology.

An ultrasound examination should follow a systematic and thorough course to ensure that all structures of the neck from clavicle to mandible are evaluated. The examination is usually performed in both the axial and longitudinal planes. In gaining experience, a beginning ultrasonographer typically develops a structured routine that ultimately leads to a comprehensive, yet expeditious, sonographic evaluation.

An appreciation of the basic physics and principles of ultrasound is important to be able to recognize the central characteristics of various tissue types. The sonographic appearance of fat is hyperechoic relative to muscle, which is hypoechoic. The cervical fascia that invests the muscles and organs of the neck is very echogenic and is seen clearly as a distinct white line that delineates structures from one another. Mucosa is

Otolaryngology – Head and Neck Surgery Service, Tripler Army Medical Center, 1 Jarrett White Road, Honolulu, HI 96859-5000, USA
E-mail address: christopher.klem@us.army.mil

Otolaryngol Clin N Am 43 (2010) 1161–1169
doi:10.1016/j.otc.2010.08.005
0030-6665/10/$ – see front matter. Published by Elsevier Inc.

oto.theclinics.com

also very echogenic and can be easily differentiated from the hypoechoic muscle that it typically overlies. Arteries are anechoic and pulsations can often be seen. Veins are also anechoic and easily compressible with pressure from the ultrasound probe.

Division of the neck into anatomic triangles based on the sternocleidomastoid, digastric, and omohyoid muscles, all of which are readily identified sonographically, creates easily recognizable landmarks on which to base a thorough examination. These triangles do not correspond exactly with the American Joint Committee on Cancer levels of the neck for cancer staging, but an examiner may do simple correlations using sonographic landmarks.[1]

The triangular-shaped area anterior to the sternocleidomastoid muscle is anatomically classified as the anterior triangle, whereas the region posterior to the muscle is termed the posterior triangle. The anterior triangle is further divided into infrahyoid and suprahyoid sections. The anterior belly of the digastric muscle subdivides the suprahyoid portion into the submandibular triangle posteriorly and submental triangle anteriorly. Below the posterior belly of the digastric muscle, the infrahyoid triangle is divided into the muscular and carotid triangles by the superior belly of the omohyoid muscle.

Borders of the posterior triangle include the sternocleidomastoid muscle anteriorly, the occiput superiorly, the clavicle inferiorly, and the trapezius muscle posteriorly. The inferior belly of the omohyoid muscle subdivides the region into the occipital triangle superiorly and the supraclavicular triangle inferiorly.

SUBMENTAL TRIANGLE (LEVEL 1A)

The anterior bellies of the right and left digastric muscles form the lateral borders of the submental triangle. The apex of the triangle is the mental symphysis, the base is the hyoid bone, and the mylohyoid muscle forms the floor. Lymph nodes are the only structures of note that reside in the submental space.

Visible via transverse imaging through the submental region are the extrinsic muscles of the tongue, including the genioglossus, geniohyoid, and hyoglossus muscles (**Fig. 1**). The sling-shaped mylohyoid muscle forms the floor of the mouth.

The lingual artery courses medial to the hyoglossus muscle, whereas the submandibular duct runs alongside the sublingual gland between the hyoglossus and more superficial mylohyoid muscle. These muscles are readily distinguished from one another, and the hyoglossus muscle can be seen contracting when the patient's tongue is moved from side to side during active ultrasonography, whereas the mylohyoid remains immobile. The hyperechoic sublingual gland is elongated and fills much of the lateral floor of mouth extending posteriorly from the submandibular gland toward the mental symphysis anteriorly.[2] An abnormally dilated submandibular duct is easily seen sonographically in the floor of the mouth, but a normal duct is less evident. The duct is differentiated from the lingual artery and vein by the lack of flow on Doppler imaging.

SUBMANDIBULAR TRIANGLE (LEVEL 1B)

The submandibular triangle is bounded by the anterior and posterior digastric bellies inferiorly and the mandible superiorly. Forming the medial border of this triangle are the hyoglossus and mylohyoid muscles. The sublingual space lies deep to the mylohyoid muscle (**Fig. 2**). The mylohyoid muscle is the key to determining whether or not pathology resides in the sublingual or submandibular space; a lesion deep to the mylohyoid arises from the sublingual space, whereas anything superficial to the muscle rests in the submandibular space.

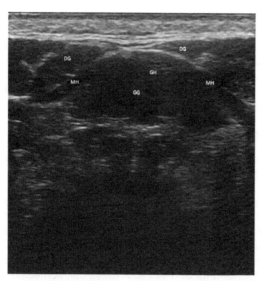

Fig. 1. Midline transverse view of the floor of mouth and tongue from the submental region. Clearly seen are the paired anterior digastric muscles (DG) and mylohyoid muscles (MH), as well as the genioglossus (GG) and geniohyoid muscles (GH).

Normal submandibular gland is homogenous and hyperechoic compared with surrounding structures.[3,4] There are also lymph nodes and fat that reside in the submandibular space, but unlike the parotid gland, there are no lymph nodes within the submandibular gland parenchyma. Any sonographic abnormalities in the gland should be considered pathologic. Because the sonographic characteristics of nerve are so similar to the surrounding tissue, the hypoglossal and lingual nerves are not usually visible.

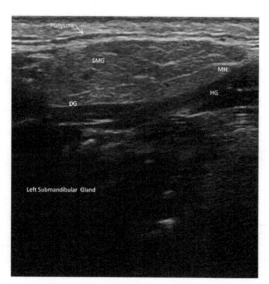

Fig. 2. The homogenous echogenicity of the submandibular gland (SMG) is clearly seen in the transverse view, along with surrounding structures, including the anterior digastric muscle (DG), mylohyoid muscle (MH), hyoglossus muscle (HG), and platysma.

The facial artery is a key feature of the submandibular space and is easily followed on its circuitous course from the external carotid artery through the triangle to the point where it crosses the body of the mandible. More superficially, the anterior facial vein and retromandibular vein are readily visualized. The retromandibular vein is an excellent landmark for distinguishing parotid space pathology posteriorly from submandibular gland disease anteriorly.[2] Wharton's duct is often visible when dilated due to distal obstruction, but a normal duct is not commonly seen.

CAROTID TRIANGLE/MUSCULAR TRIANGLE (LEVELS 2, 3, 4)

Inferior to the posterior belly of the digastric is the carotid triangle, bounded anteriorly by the superior belly of the omohyoid muscle and posteriorly by the sternocleidomastoid muscle.

Immediately evident sonographically are the vascular structures of the carotid sheath, including the carotid artery and internal jugular vein. Especially in this region, color flow Doppler helps distinguish blood vessels from other structures. It is important to scan in both the axial and longitudinal planes because blood vessels are round when the transducer is axial and appear as an anechoic linear structure when the transducer is longitudinal (**Fig. 3**). The vagus nerve can sometimes be seen as a dot on axial imaging or as a hypoechoic line medial to the carotid artery on longitudinal imaging (**Fig. 4A**).[5]

The internal jugular vein is typically lateral and slightly superficial to the artery. There is variability in the size of the vein, with the right side typically larger than the left. The vein is easily compressible with gentle pressure from the ultrasound transducer, whereas the carotid artery is not. When a patient performs a Valsalva maneuver, the vein also dilates (see **Fig. 4**).

More superiorly in this region, the internal and external carotid arteries, as well as the bifurcation of the artery, are readily seen deep and anterior to the hypoechoic sternocleidomastoid muscle. Unlike the compressible internal jugular vein, the carotid artery is pulsatile and does not compress easily or change size with Valsalva. Also common is a posterior enhancement effect, an artifact that is present when the distal reflected echoes behind an area of low attenuation (in this case, anechoic blood in the

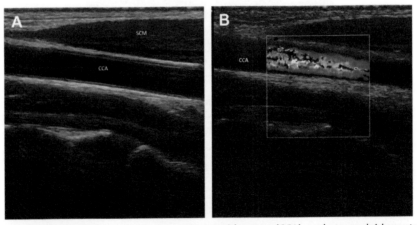

Fig. 3. Longitudinal view of the common carotid artery (CCA) and sternocleidomastoid muscle (SCM) (A). Color flow Doppler in the sagittal plane confirms that a structure is vascular in nature (B).

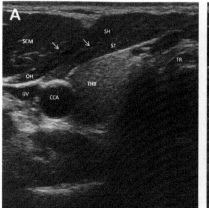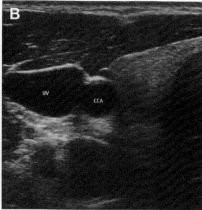

Fig. 4. Transverse image of the right thyroid lobe. Note the compressed internal jugular vein (IJV) lateral to the common carotid artery (CCA) (*A*) compared with the distended internal jugular vein (*B*) when the patient performs a Valsalva maneuver. Also well seen are the thyroid gland (THY), tracheal rings (TR), the sternocleidomastoid muscle (SCM), and the omohyoid (OH), sternohyoid (SH), and sternothyroid (ST) muscles all separated by a fascial layer (*arrows*).

lumen of the carotid artery) appear enhanced compared with adjacent tissue. External carotid branches can often be followed distally from their origin. The carotid bifurcation is at approximately the level of the hyoid bone and marks the lower limit of level 2.

Scanning inferiorly from the carotid bifurcation, the common carotid artery, internal jugular vein, and sternocleidomastoid muscle are the major structures in the field of view. The inferior border of level 3 and the carotid triangle is the superior belly of the omohyoid muscle, a hypoechoic structure that runs obliquely from posteroinferior to anterosuperior across the superficial aspect of the internal jugular vein.

Lymph nodes are commonly seen in the carotid and muscular triangles. Nonpathologic lymph nodes are oval or kidney bean shaped, hypoechoic, and have a central fatty hilum that is echogenic (**Fig. 5**). Running through the hilum are afferent and efferent lymphatics as well as arterial and venous supply that can often be seen on color flow Doppler. The size criteria for what is considered a pathologic lymph node is controversial; many use 1.0 cm as the upper limit of normal for otherwise ordinary-appearing lymph nodes, except for the jugulodigastric node, which is given an upper limit of 1.5 cm. Regardless of size, in the presence of a known malignancy, a lymph node without a normal sonographic appearance should be considered suspicious for metastatic spread.

The muscular triangle, which corresponds to level 4, is bordered superiorly by the superior belly of the omohyoid, posteriorly by the sternocleidomastoid muscle, and anteriorly by the sternohyoid muscle. Carotid sheath structures, the anterior scalene muscle, and lymphatics are the prevalent structures in the muscular triangle. This muscle originates from the transverse processes of the cervical spine, runs deep to the carotid sheath, and attaches to the first rib. Inferiorly, the common carotid artery can be followed to its junction with the subclavian artery by aiming the transducer cephalad.

POSTERIOR TRIANGLE (LEVEL 5)

Initially, the posterior triangle can be a challenging region to understand sonographically. The region is superficial and is comprised primarily of muscles around the border

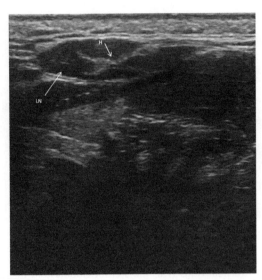

Fig. 5. Benign lymph node. Note the oblong, hypoechoic nature of the lymph node (LN) and the hyperechoic, fatty hilum (H) that includes the vascular pedicle (*arrows*).

and the floor. Forming the deep boundary of the triangle are the scalene, levator scapulae, and splenius capitis muscles. The inferior belly of the omohyoid muscle delineates the occipital triangle above from the supraclavicular triangle below. Residing in the cervical fascia superficial to the floor are the spinal accessory nerve and lymph nodes, fat, the brachial plexus, and the transverse cervical artery and vein. The spinal accessory nerve is difficult to see on ultrasound.

Inferior to the inferior belly of the omohyoid muscle, the supraclavicular triangle is also bounded by the trapezius muscle posteriorly, the sternocleidomastoid muscle anteriorly, and the clavicle inferiorly. The subclavian vein is often seen posterior to the clavicle. Emerging from the lateral aspect of the scalene muscles, the brachial plexus can be seen as rounded hypoechoic structures on axial imaging.

THYROID/PARATHYROID

High-resolution ultrasound of the thyroid gland reveals remarkable detail about the gland and surrounding structures. Coupled with the superficial location in the anterior neck, this is an excellent region for beginning ultrasonographers to gain experience and confidence.

Normal thyroid parenchyma is hyperechoic and homogenous compared with the relatively hypoechoic strap muscles, the sternothyroid and sternohyoid, that border the gland anteriorly. The cervical fascia investing the muscles and the thyroid gland is echogenic and appears as a thin white line (see **Fig. 4**). Interruption of the fascia surrounding the gland should alert an examiner to the possibility of extrathyroidal extension by a malignancy.

There is commonly slight asymmetry between the right and left thyroid lobes, both in size and location. Although present in approximately 80% of people, the pyramidal lobe is not commonly seen because of its small diameter.

The trachea lies posterior to the thyroid and the common carotid arteries border the gland laterally on each side. The esophagus is typically seen inferiorly, deep to the left thyroid lobe.

Both the superior and inferior thyroid arteries can be traced from their origins at the external carotid artery and thyrocervical trunk, respectively, to the gland. The inferior thyroid artery passes deep to the common carotid artery and where the vessel enters the gland is an excellent marker for the depth of the recurrent laryngeal nerve. Color flow Doppler is essential to aid in differentiating blood vessels from cystic thyroid pathology.

Ultrasound evaluation for parathyroids is usually done as a localization study preoperatively in the setting of primary hyperparathyroidism. Normal parathyroid glands are rarely visible sonographically. The superior glands are more predictably found in close proximity to the cricothyroid joint, whereas the inferior glands have a more variable location.

LARYNX/TRACHEA/ESOPHAGUS (LEVEL 6)

Despite being air filled, the structures of the larynx and trachea lie superficially in the neck and have good inherent soft tissue contrast making them ideally suited for visualization with ultrasound.

In the midline of the neck deep to the thyroid gland, the cartilaginous tracheal rings and cricoid are useful landmarks in both the axial and longitudinal planes (**Fig. 6**). The cricoid cartilage forms a complete ring and is the most cephalad portion of the trachea. Below the cricoid, the first 5 to 6 tracheal rings can be seen with gentle neck extension. Several reports of the use of high-resolution ultrasound to assist with visualization of the trachea during percutaneous tracheotomy are published.[6,7]

The larynx lies between the cricoid cartilage inferiorly and the hyoid bone superiorly. Variable ossification of the laryngeal framework, including the thyroid and cricoid cartilages, causes the sonographic appearance of the larynx to differ significantly between patients. The thyroid, cricoid, and arytenoid cartilages are all echogenic, whereas the intrinsic muscles of the larynx appear hypoechoic. The laryngeal mucosa is also hyperechoic, in contrast to the anechoic intraluminal air column. The differing acoustic characteristics allow differentiation of these structures. Fat in the pre-epiglottic space

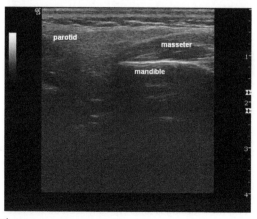

Fig. 6. Parotid gland.

is echogenic, whereas the cartilage of the epiglottis is hypoechoic. This region is best visualized via the thyrohyoid membrane.[5]

Usually to the left of the trachea, the esophagus has a characteristic echogenic center of air and saliva with a hypoechoic muscular rim, often described as a bull's eye or target (**Fig. 7**). When a patient swallows, the hyperechoic esophageal center dilates actively and then returns to the resting state.[2]

PAROTID SPACE

The boundaries of the parotid space are the external auditory canal superiorly, the masseter muscle anteriorly, and the mandible and medial pterygoid muscle medially. The posterior digastric muscle is the inferior border of the parotid space and forms the superior boundary of the carotid triangle below.[5]

Normal parotid tissue is sonographically similar to submandibular gland and is hyperechoic and homogenous. When scanning, areas in the gland that are hypoechoic suggest abnormal pathology.[8]

Multiple lymph nodes normally reside in the gland and may be evident on ultrasound examination. Although the facial nerve itself is not visible sonographically, the retromandibular vein travels in a craniocaudad direction and its location is a reliable approximation for the depth of the facial nerve (see **Fig. 6**). Arbitrary delineation of superficial and deep lobes of the parotid gland can be made with the retromandibular vein as the reference. Although a dilated parotid (Stensen's) duct is readily sonographically apparent, a normal duct can sometimes be seen as an echogenic line within the superficial lobe. When an accessory parotid lobe is present, it typically lies along the course of the parotid duct lateral to the masseter muscle.[2]

ANATOMY KNOWLEDGE ESSENTIAL FOR EFFECTIVE ULTRASOUND

Ultrasound is an effective instrument for otolaryngology–head and neck surgeons. A thorough knowledge of head and neck anatomy, as well as the sonographic

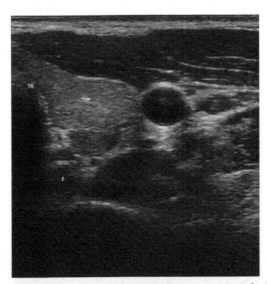

Fig. 7. In the lower neck, the esophagus (E) is typically seen on the left side adjacent to the trachea (TR) and deep to the left thyroid lobe (THY).

appearance of normal anatomic structures in this complex region, is essential. The comprehensive familiarity with head and neck anatomy gained through surgery makes ultrasound especially suited to use by surgeons.

REFERENCES

1. Agur AM. Grant's atlas of anatomy. 12th edition. Baltimore (MD): Williams & Wilkins; 2008.
2. Evans RM. Anatomy and technique. In: Ahuja A, Evans R, editors. Practical head and neck ultrasound. London: Greenwich Medical Media Ltd; 2003. p. 1–16.
3. Alyas F, Lewis K, Williams M, et al. Diseases of the submandibular gland as demonstrated using high resolution ultrasound. Br J Radiol 2005;78:362–9.
4. Howlett DC, Alyas F, Wong KT, et al. Sonographic assessment of the submandibular space. Clin Radiol 2004;59:1070–8.
5. Gourin CG, Orlorr LA. Normal head and neck ultrasound anatomy. In: Orloff LA, editor. Head and neck ultrasonography. San Diego (CA): Plural Publishing Inc; 2008. p. 39–68.
6. Bertram S, Emshoff R, Norer B. Ultrasonographic anatomy of the anterior neck: Implications for tracheostomy. J Oral Maxillofac Surg 1995;53:1420–4.
7. Muhammad JK, Patton DW, Evans RM, et al. Percutaneous dilational tracheostomy (PDT) under ultrasound guidance. Br J Oral Maxillofac Surg 1999;37:309–11.
8. Zajkowski P, Jakubowski W, Bialek EJ, et al. Pleomorphic adenoma and adenolymphoma in ultrasonography. Eur J Ultrasound 2000;12:23–9.

Interpretation of Ultrasound

Robert A. Sofferman, MD

KEYWORDS

- Ultrasound interpretation • Pathologic correlation
- Sonographic artifacts • Head and neck ultrasonography

A thorough knowledge of head and neck anatomy is critical to defining what are normal and abnormal findings on high-resolution ultrasound. At first, the transverse and sagittal orientations of the transducer can be confusing to the operator. The best way to overcome this problem is to select concentrated areas of the neck and identify as many normal structures as possible within that area. Instead of using a Doppler whenever a suspect blood vessel is identified, the operator will better understand relationships by tracing as much as possible the course of the vessel in gray scale both in transverse and sagittal planes. The transition from normal anatomy and a sound knowledge of scanning artifacts will serve as the best foundation for properly interpreting pathologic conditions.

ULTRASOUND INTERPRETATION IN HEAD AND NECK PATHOLOGY

The beauty of ultrasound is that the examination process occurs in real time with the examiner learning how to merge the various planes of view into a dynamic 3-dimensional image. There is no substitute for the circumstance where the operator/managing clinician is performing this dynamic examination while constructing a concurrent differential diagnosis. A technician who does not possess the knowledge base of head and neck pathology is quite limited in this aspect of ultrasonography. However, radiologic technicians and radiologists are well educated about standardizing the examination process. This redundancy from one examination to the next is valuable in comparison of normal with abnormal structure, and it lessens the likelihood of omissions.

The otolaryngologist who performs office-based ultrasound must avoid cutting corners in defense of time to maintain a proper standard and to avoid overlooking a key portion of the examination. As an example, it is easy to omit a proper survey of lymph node basins when concentrating on a thyroid nodule and, of course, both elements may be linked and are important to examine in the same ultrasound

Division of Otolaryngology, University of Vermont School of Medicine, Fletcher Allen Health Care, ACC West Pavilion 4th Floor, 111 Colchester Avenue, Burlington, Vermont 05401, USA
E-mail address: robert.sofferman@vtmednet.org

Otolaryngol Clin N Am 43 (2010) 1171–1202
doi:10.1016/j.otc.2010.08.008
0030-6665/10/$ – see front matter © 2010 Elsevier Inc. All rights reserved.

procedure. Conversely, a thyroid examination should be part of every head and neck ultrasound procedure. Thyroid pathology is common and malignancies can be occult and asymptomatic. In a similar manner, lymphadenopathy alone may not be as meaningful as lymphadenopathy in conjunction with an irregular thyroid nodule containing microcalcifications.

This article is constructed to present some of the pathologic conditions that affect the salivary glands, soft tissues, lymph nodes, thyroid and parathyroid glands, esophagus, vascular structures, congenital cysts, and even mandibular relationships. The content provides the physician with information and representative images of the more common conditions involving the head and neck. Some of this information may also be covered elsewhere in this publication, but it is presented here as a systems overview and stepping point for further in-depth study. High-resolution ultrasound is the best modality for detailing pathology of the thyroid gland before fine-needle aspiration cytology. An enlarged parotid gland is often mystifying at initial history and physical examination, but the added advantage of concurrent ultrasound usually allows the clinician to understand the problem and direct earlier proper management.

Skin and Subcutaneous Tissues

High-resolution transducers in the range of 10 to 12 MHz provide good detail of the skin and subcutaneous tissues. If one has access to even higher frequency probes, ie, 17 MHz, the image detail can be stunning. One very helpful use of the ultrasound examination of a skin-related process is to differentiate cellulitis from abscess, especially in children. A cellulitic process is diffuse and edema of the tissues can be identified on ultrasound. In contrast, an abscess is usually a discrete hypoechoic to anechoic area that may extend deep to the subcutaneous plane (**Fig. 1**). A foreign body can usually be identified even if it is not ferromagnetic or may not demonstrate on conventional soft tissue radiograph. Fistulous tracts are hypoechoic channels that usually can be traced to the site of origin (**Fig. 2**). If the fistula arises from the skin surface, the tract can be easily traced and the condition properly identified. A fistula arising from the aerodigestive tract that extends into the subcutaneous tissues or thyroid (fourth branchial pouch sinus) may be traceable on ultrasound (**Fig. 3**).

Frequently, ultrasound is the initial study as part of a more comprehensive imaging profile. In many instances, it can suffice as the only requisite study. A sebaceous cyst is usually properly identified and characterized by physical examination alone, but it is instructive to demonstrate its sonographic characteristics (**Fig. 4**A, B). It is usually seen at the level of the dermis and can extend by pressure enlargement to involve the subcutaneous level. The mass is discrete and well-encapsulated and the contained sebum does not produce as homogeneous an image as a fluid-filled cyst. Posterior enhancement is present to some degree. Lipomas are common and usually arise from the subcutaneous adipose tissues (**Fig. 5**A). They have a soft, somewhat compressible physical characteristic, but occasionally differentiation from a lymph node can be difficult. Fine-needle aspiration without ultrasound guidance will be nondiagnostic and the lipocytes will be misinterpreted as contaminants during the penetration process. The ultrasonographic features of a lipoma are virtually diagnostic. The overall structure is ovoid and somewhat discrete from the surrounding subcutaneous tissues. Horizontal hyperechoic lines are its hallmark, probably representative of the connective tissue bands that compartmentalize the lipoma. Power Doppler confirms the avascular nature of the mass. Lipomas can be found wherever there is adipose tissue. An example of a parotid lipoma is demonstrated (see **Fig. 5**B). The sonographic

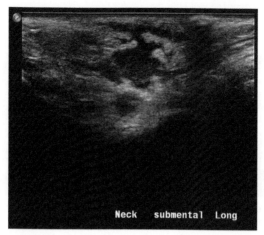

Fig. 1. Subcutaneous abscess.

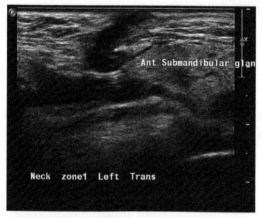

Fig. 2. A fistula from the mandible to submandibular skin is associated in this circumstance with a prior dental implant.

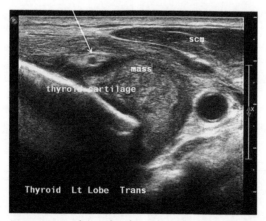

Fig. 3. An inflammatory mass overlying the thyroid cartilage or within the left thyroid lobe can be secondary to a fistula arising from the apex of the pyriform sinus. The arrow points to the actual sinus tract.

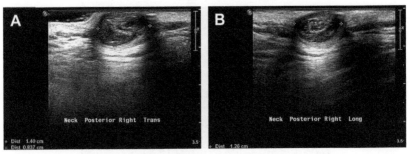

Fig. 4. (*A, B*) Sebaceous cyst in transverse and longitudinal planes. Note that the epicenter of the cyst is at 5 mm from the skin surface.

features are so typical that the diagnosis can be established on ultrasound study alone.

Salivary Glands

The normal parotid and submaxillary glands have the same ground-glass appearance on ultrasound. Whereas the submaxillary gland is relatively discrete and its dimensions easy to measure, the parotid gland is more difficult to define. Both glands contain large, intermediate, and small ducts and share an intimate relationship with surrounding lymph nodes. In fact, subcapsular lymphadenopathy is usually identified within the parenchyma of the parotid gland. Of all studies to investigate parotid

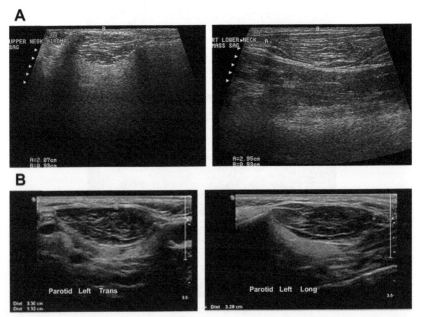

Fig. 5. (*A*) An ovoid subcutaneous mass with horizontal striations is typical of a lipoma. (*B*) The same horizontal striations are indicative of a lipoma in this parotid gland.

pathology, ultrasound is an efficient and cost-effective modality with no radiation exposure. In addition to the initial study, it permits an easy method to efficiently track an inflammatory process over time.

Obstructing Calculus

In this condition, the ductal system will be ecstatic (**Fig. 6**A). The examiner may not be certain whether these conduits are of ductal or vascular origin; the Doppler assessment clarifies the findings with certainty (see **Fig. 6**B). A careful inspection of the ductal system distal to the gland hilum may reveal a discrete hyperechoic density that also demonstrates posterior shadowing artifact (**Fig. 7**). Occasionally, multiple stones may be seen in the duct system, and if they are smaller than the walls of the obstructed duct, the ultrasound waves may cause them to move or vibrate. This can be seen on the real-time images and archived with cine loops (**Fig. 8**).

Diffuse Parotitis

The gland may be inflamed with evidence or obstruction to the main duct system. In this circumstance, there may be edema or areas of heterogeneity throughout the gland and the gland itself is enlarged (**Fig. 9**). It is always a good idea in this circumstance to examine and measure the salivary glands in question bilaterally to compare the normal with abnormal architecture and dimensions.

Sjogren's Syndrome

Lymphoepithelial lesions of the parotid glands have a very distinct image characteristic. The histopathology demonstrates discrete areas throughout the gland that resemble germinal centers in a lymph node (**Fig. 10**). This same appearance can be identified on ultrasound with multiple discrete hypoechoic islands throughout the entire gland. This same echo-appearance is noted in Mikulicz disease and recurrent parotitis of childhood.

Parotid Cysts

A single parotid cyst may represent a focal obstruction of a smaller proximal duct, or as a congenital anomaly (first branchial cleft cyst). These cysts are discrete, rounded, anechoic, thinly encapsulated, and demonstrate bright posterior enhancement (**Fig. 11**). Parotid cysts, either single or multiple, may indicate HIV disease.

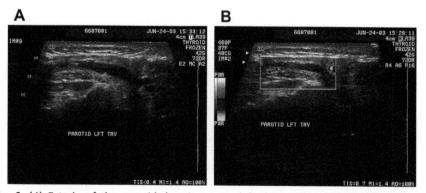

Fig. 6. (*A*) Ectasia of the parotid duct is a typical finding with an obstructing calculus. (*B*) Ectasia of the duct system can be differentiated from a vessel with Doppler assessment.

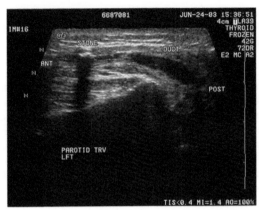

Fig. 7. A distal calculus is identified with posterior shadowing artifact.

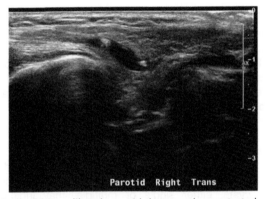

Fig. 8. Multiple calculi within a dilated parotid duct are demonstrated.

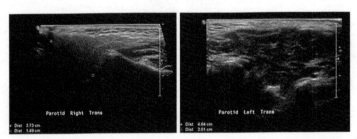

Fig. 9. Diffuse heterogeneous hypoechoic areas within the symptomatic gland are compared with a ground glass appearance of the opposite normal parotid.

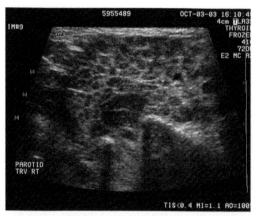

Fig. 10. In Sjogren's syndrome the gland is replaced with a diffuse "honey-combed" appearance.

Occasionally, the cyst will contain proteinaceous debris, which presents on ultrasound as discrete punctate areas throughout the cyst (**Fig. 12**). In real time, this debris may demonstrate vibratory movement from the transmitted sound waves.

Tumor

A mass within the parenchyma of either the submaxillary or parotid gland cannot be classified with certainty without cytologic confirmation; however, there are sonographic findings that may suggest the likelihood of malignancy. The most worrisome abnormalities are irregular ill-defined borders of the mass (**Fig. 13**) with a surrounding normal gland, infiltration of the skin or adjacent muscles, and clear-cut malignant adenopathy of the upper neck in association with a parotid mass. Conversely, a very discrete mass with sharply marginated borders may demonstrate some irregularity in knoblike but confined projections. This type of mass may demonstrate

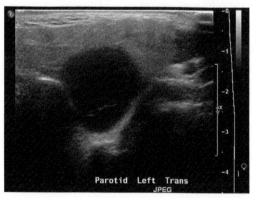

Fig. 11. As with all fluid-filled cysts, those in the parotid have a rounded appearance, are sharply marginated, and demonstrate posterior enhancement.

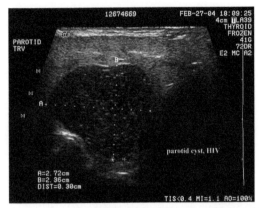

Fig. 12. Proteinaceous debris may fill the interior of the cyst. When multiple, HIV should be suspected.

a hypoechoic uniform echo architecture and posterior enhancement artifact, which usually is supportive of a cyst.

The one solid tumor that demonstrates posterior enhancement is a benign mixed tumor (**Fig. 14**). A Warthin tumor may demonstrate characteristics of a cyst, but generally it is not as homogeneous as a mixed tumor and does not demonstrate discrete projections. Parotid malignancies such as adenoid cystic, mucoepidermoid, and acinic cell carcinomas often do not demonstrate specific sonographic features. Thus, fine-needle aspiration cytology is mandatory for any salivary gland mass.

Occasionally, the precise tissue type cannot be determined; the cytopathologist may be able to diagnose only malignancy, but not much more. Ultrasound-guided core biopsy (16- or 18-gauge) is an excellent adjunctive procedure in this circumstance to allow the pathologist to render a precise diagnosis before surgical intervention. Intraoperative frozen section may similarly plague the pathologist, especially if

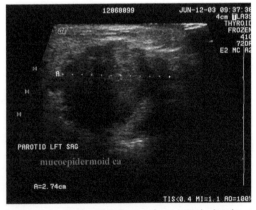

Fig. 13. Parotid masses with irregular margins to the normal gland are strongly suspicious for malignancy.

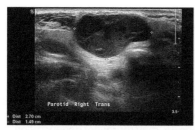
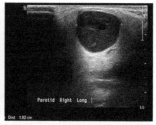

Fig. 14. Pleomorphic adenomas have smooth, sharp margins and may have projections that are still encapsulated. This is the only parotid tumor that demonstrates striking posterior enhancement.

critical decisions regarding the facial nerve depend on accurate histopathology. A diffuse infiltrative process may be identified as parotid lymphoma, which can be partially characterized with fine-needle aspiration cytology and flow cytometry. Again, core biopsy under ultrasound guidance may be all that is required to precisely identify the lymphoma type and direct appropriate treatment.

Patients with benign mixed tumors who have either tumor spill at surgery or improper management with incisional biopsy are at risk for multiple nodular recurrence. Ultrasound is an excellent modality to carefully map each of the recurrent nodules, either before revision surgery or intraoperatively (**Fig. 15**).

CERVICAL CYSTS

Cystic lesions of the head and neck do not have the same uniform etiology. Some arise from congenital connections with the aerodigestive tract and others develop from obstructing ductal structures or ill-defined degenerative processes within a solid organ or mass.

Thyroglossal Duct Cysts

Although usually midline in location, thyroglossal duct cysts can present as masses off the midline over the thyroid ala, at the thyroid notch and thyrohyoid membrane, and

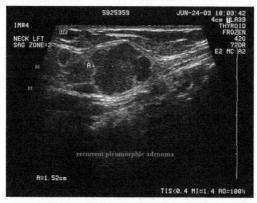

Fig. 15. Recurrent pleomorphic adenomas may be multiple and these can be carefully mapped with ultrasound before revision surgery or as an intraoperative modality.

even in the submental triangle. These cysts may be single or multiloculated but always demonstrate the same characteristics: (1) discrete capsule, (2) anechoic echo architecture, and (3) posterior enhancement (**Fig. 16**).

Branchial Cleft Cyst

Second arch cysts are characteristically located at or near the carotid bifurcation and have the same sonographic characteristics as described for the thyroglossal duct cyst. A cyst in the upper neck, often in zone IIa, may represent degeneration of a metastatic squamous cell carcinoma to a lymph node (**Fig. 17**). Occasionally a cyst will be identified on the left side of the neck in zone III or IV and may be associated with recurrent cellulitis or thyroiditis. Frequently, no discrete cyst is identified, only inflammation and occasionally abscess formation. Careful inspection of the area lateral to the thyroid ala and cricoid cartilage may demonstrate a fistulous tract, suggesting the likelihood of a fourth branchial pouch fistula arising from the pyriform sinus (**Fig. 18**A, B). Occasionally, fistulae can arise from the lateral wall of the hypopharynx. One clue to the proper condition may be entrapped food or vegetable matter, which produces an unusual reflective pattern (see **Fig. 18**C). The ultrasound simply allows the clinician to suspect the diagnosis; esophagogram or contrast-enhanced CT swallow defines the pathology with best accuracy (see **Fig. 18**D).

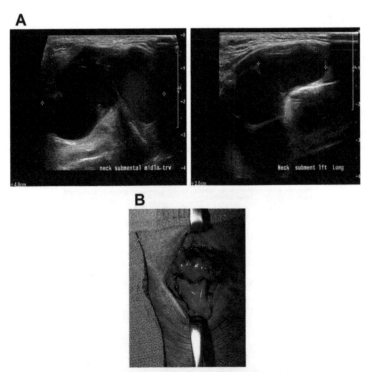

Fig. 16. (*A*) These congenital cysts are closely applied to the thyroid notch and a large cyst is identified over the thyrohyoid region in this sagittal view. (*B*) The operative findings are included for comparison with the actual thyroglossal duct cyst.

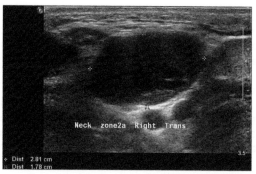

Fig. 17. This cyst in zone II is actually a necrotic lymph node completely replaced by metastatic squamous cell carcinoma.

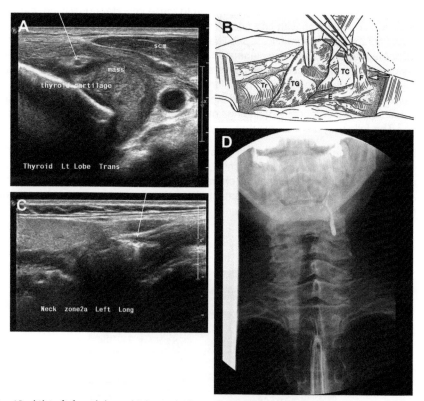

Fig. 18. (A) Left fourth branchial pouch sinus. The arrow points to the sinus tract that leads to an inflammatory mass. (B) Artist's rendition of fourth branchial pouch sinus. (C) Left pharyngeal pouch with entrapped food indicated by refractile sound artifacts. Arrow directs attention to the area of the pouch and refractile food particles. (D) Subsequent barium swallow demonstrates the pouch.

Ranula

A cystic mass in zone I either in the submental region or somewhat lateral may either be superficial to the mylohyoid muscle or demonstrate an extension posteriorly adjacent or deep to the submandibular gland. When the cyst extends posteriorly, it is deep to the mylohyoid muscle (**Fig. 19**). Doppler can be used to confirm the avascular nature of this structure. Needle aspiration confirms the texture and color of the fluid as of salivary origin. An amylase analysis of the fluid may be obtained to confirm a diagnosis of ranula. A similar cystic lesion that often has septations and is demonstrated to be macrocystic may reveal straw-colored fluid on aspiration. If cytology demonstrates abundant lymphocytes, the diagnosis of lymphoangioma is confirmed.

LYMPH NODES

Understanding the anatomy of a normal lymph node and its differentiation from one with metastasis or lymphoma is one of the most important advantages of head and neck ultrasound. In addition to the accurate identification of a pathologic node that may not be evident on palpation often has important therapeutic implications. It is critical to identify significant adenopathy but also to accurately describe its precise location into an appropriate neck zone. In addition to these important qualifying features, ultrasound in conjunction with fine-needle aspiration cytology provides accurate and relatively noninvasive diagnostic capabilities. Finally, simple chemical assessment of the aspirate may allow definitive diagnostic information, ie, thyroglobulin identification in a node confirms the presence of metastatic thyroid carcinoma and a node positive for calcitonin confirms metastatic medullary cancer of the thyroid.

There is no single sonographic characteristic of a lymph node that defines malignancy, but rather a composite of findings may allow the clinician to be strongly suspicious.[1] The following are features that may suggest malignant lymphadenopathy:

1. Large size—The average lymph node is 1 to 1.5 cm in greatest dimension. Upper cervical nodes, especially in the child or adolescent, may be 2 or 3 times this average size but will retain other characteristics of normalcy. Most nodes that are abnormally large, ie, 4 cm in greatest dimension also demonstrate other abnormalities (**Fig. 20**).

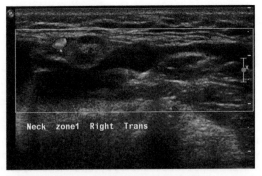

Fig. 19. A plunging ranula extends from the submental region posteriorly to the submandibular gland where the ranula has traversed the mylohyoid.

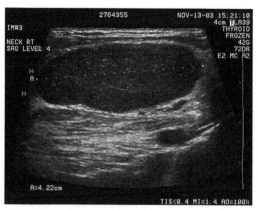

Fig. 20. Large lymphomatous lymph node.

2. Rounded shape—The average benign node is at least twice as long as it is wide. Exceptions to this measurement relationship are submental nodes that are often round rather than ovoid in shape. Lymphomatous nodes are often large and rounded (**Fig. 21**). The S/L ratio is an abbreviation sometimes used to illustrate this point. A short/long ratio of less than 0.5 is generally regarded as a normal value.
3. Irregular margin—Nodes that are irregular are also usually larger than average. The capsule of the node may be ill defined and incomplete when malignant cells extend into perinodal soft tissue or adjacent muscle. This is one of the most significant ultrasonographic features of malignancy (**Fig. 22**).
4. Multiple nodes—Nodes that are matted together or multiple in one or more zones are likely to be pathologic. Inflammatory conditions such as tuberculosis or cat scratch disease may demonstrate these features. Lymphomatous nodes are often multiple in number (**Fig. 23**).
5. Loss of hilar architecture—The nodal hilum is usually seen in a normal lymph node. This is a central hyperechoic linear structure that locates the artery, emerging vein,

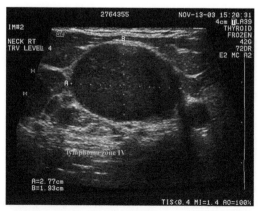

Fig. 21. In a rounded lymph node, transverse and sagittal dimensions are nearly equivalent.

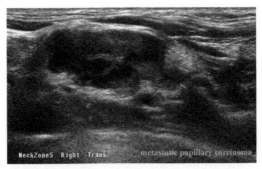

Fig. 22. An irregular border of a lymph node suggests extracapsular extension.

and efferent lymphatics of the node (**Fig. 24**A, B). Absence of this hilar line may suggest that the node is replaced by an infiltrative process. In hyperplastic lymphadenopathy, the hilum is usually preserved and the vasculature may be more evident than normal with power Doppler (see **Fig. 24**C). The normal hilum may be quite thick in structure or even occupy a significant portion of the nodal substance.

6. Peripheral vascularity—Every enlarged or suspect node should be examined with Doppler. Depending on the Doppler resolution of the ultrasound machine as well as dimension of the actual vessels, the hilar vasculature may not be apparent even in a normal node. If the axial hilar vessels are identified, the node is normal and not neoplastic. If there is peripheral hypervascularity surrounding the node or transnodal multiple vessels, angiogenic vessels may be responsible, indicative of metastatic malignancy (**Fig. 25**A, B).

7. Echogenicity—Homogeneous echo architecture in a large rounded node may reflect the "fish flesh" gross appearance seen in lymphomatous nodes (**Fig. 26**). Any cystic anechoic nodes are suspicious for metastatic papillary carcinoma (**Fig. 27**). Areas of anechoic echogenicity within a node may suggest necrosis and metastatic malignancy (**Fig. 28**).

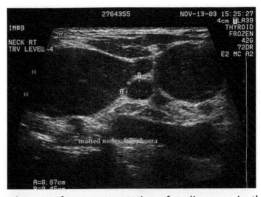

Fig. 23. Multiple nodes are often representative of malignancy, in this instance a non-Hodgkin lymphoma.

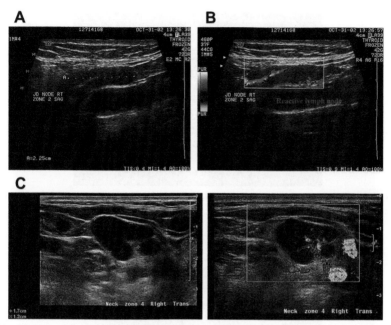

Fig. 24. (*A*) When identified, a hilar line is characteristic of a benign lymph node. (*B*) Power Doppler demonstrates the axial vessel along the hilum in this same node. (*C*) A round or large node may simply be hyperplastic and not malignant. When a well-defined hilar vasculature is identified, malignancy is less likely.

8. Calcification—Coarse calcifications are seen in a variety of benign conditions and are typically discrete areas of hyperechogenicity with posterior shadowing artifact (**Fig. 29**). These calcifications are common in both benign and malignant thyroid lesions but are uncommon in lymph nodes. Microcalcifications are punctate areas of hyperechoic signal, which in contrast to coarse calcifications do not produce posterior shadowing (**Fig. 30**A, B). When in lymph nodes, they commonly represent

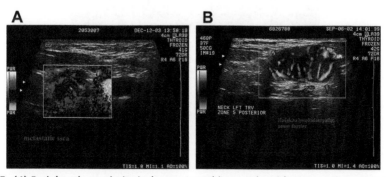

Fig. 25. (*A*) Peripheral vascularity is demonstrated in a node with metastatic squamous cell carcinoma. (*B*) Trans-nodal vessels are seen in gray scale in this lymphomatous node.

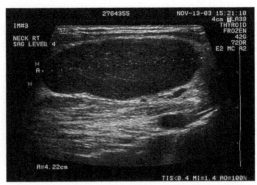

Fig. 26. Homogeneous appearance of a node with non-Hodgkin lymphoma. No axial vascularity can be identified.

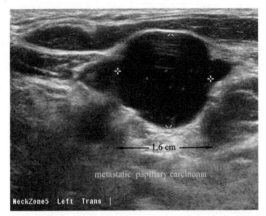

Fig. 27. This cystic node with microcalcifications is typical of metastatic papillary carcinoma.

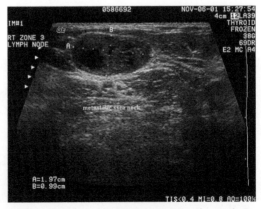

Fig. 28. Anechoic areas in a lymph node suggest necrosis. This node is replaced by areas of metastatic squamous cell carcinoma.

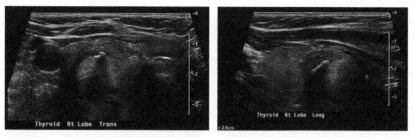

Fig. 29. Coarse thyroid calcifications are densely hyperechoic and demonstrate posterior shadowing artifact.

metastatic papillary carcinoma (see **Fig. 30**C). They may also be identified in medullary carcinoma (**Fig. 31**). Of all sonographic characteristics, microcalcifications may be the most suggestive of metastatic papillary carcinoma to lymph nodes.

The aforementioned nodal characteristics are general guidelines. Most malignant nodes do not demonstrate all of these elements, but when several of these features

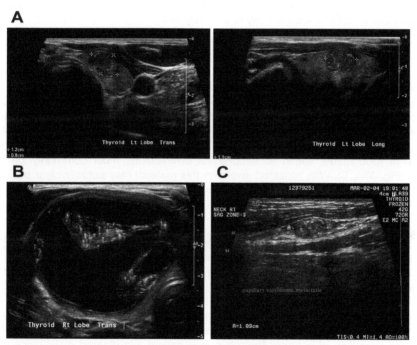

Fig. 30. (A) Microcalcifications are multiple punctuate hyperlucencies that do not show posterior shadowing. (B) When comet tails extend from punctate hyperlucencies, these are not microcalcifications, although the resemblance is close. They represent crystalline aggregates of colloid and are always indicative of a benign condition. (C) Microcalcifications in a lymph node indicate metastatic papillary carcinoma.

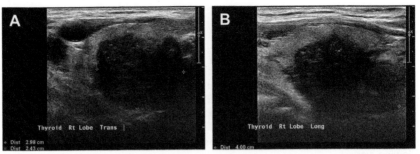

Fig. 31. (*A, B*) Papillary carcinoma of the thyroid demonstrating a few microcalcifications. The anatomic correlates to punctate microcalcifications are psammoma bodies demonstrated in the histologic image.

are identified, suspicion for malignant adenopathy should become a clinical consideration. A recent study by Liao and colleagues[2] nicely illustrates this point. Nodes are assessed for patient age, S/L ratio, internal echogenic characteristics, and vascular pattern and each element is given a weighted score. Cervical nodes are determined to be malignant with scores of equal or greater than 7 with a sensitivity of 100.0%, specificity of 88.0%, and overall accuracy of 90.1% when compared with actual histology. This scoring system recognizes that no single element defines a malignant node but selects a few key sonographic features that as a composite accurately predict that a cervical node is likely to be malignant.

ESOPHAGUS

The esophagus is a hypoechoic circular structure visualized to the posterolateral aspect of the left lobe of the thyroid on transverse images (**Fig. 32**A). Sagittal views may nicely demonstrate the longitudinal fibers of the esophagus (see **Fig. 32**B). Occasionally, the esophagus is located to the right of the thyroid. A hypoechoic mass adjacent to the esophagus, usually noted on the sagittal view, may demonstrate parallel bright transmitted lines in a "sunburst" pattern. These represent artifacts from vegetable or food matter within an esophageal diverticulum, most commonly Zenker type (**Fig. 33**A, B). With repeated swallows this material may actually clear partially or completely (see **Fig. 33**C, D). Pharyngeal pouches may demonstrate the same refractive food material as demonstrated.

VASCULAR SYSTEM

Dynamic evaluation of a vascular system is one of the most important attributes of cervical high-resolution ultrasound. With a simple touch of a "Doppler button," the examiner can evaluate vascular anatomy, vascular flow pattern of small structures such as lymph nodes, the presence or absence of flow in major structures such as the internal jugular vein, and determine whether a lesion or tumor is of vascular origin. Inflammatory internal jugular vein thrombosis can be identified quite readily (**Fig. 34**) and the suspicion of a tumor thrombus in a patient with thyroid malignancy can have important therapeutic ramifications (**Fig. 35**A, B, C, D). Thyroid nodules are frequently identified incidentally in the course of a carotid vascular study. Conversely, carotid atherosclerosis at the bifurcation may be identified during the course of head and neck ultrasound stimulating appropriate clinical referral (**Fig. 36**).

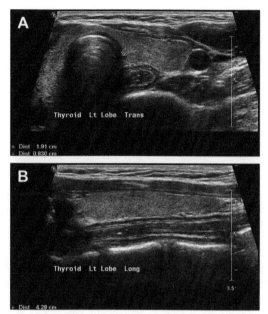

Fig. 32. (*A*) The normal esophagus is a rounded structure in transverse view, usually noted on the left side of the trachea. (*B*) In sagittal view the esophagus is a uniform longitudinal structure alongside the thyroid gland.

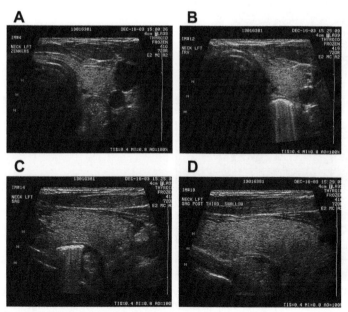

Fig. 33. (*A*) A Zenker diverticulum is suspected when the esophagus seems enlarged and contains material that demonstrates bizarre refractile artifacts. (*B, C, D*) With sequential swallows, the refractile food particles may clear.

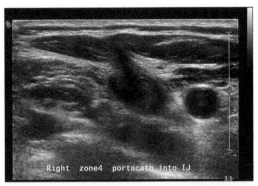

Fig. 34. The internal jugular vein does not illuminate with Doppler when there is thrombosis. In this circumstance, a central-line catheter in the vein for administration of chemotherapy is responsible for the thrombosis.

Cystic lesions of the parotid or zone I may demonstrate multiple septations. This lesion may be either a lymphangioma or hemangioma and Doppler can easily differentiate them. The hemangioma has large vascular spaces between the septae and lymphangioma demonstrates a lack of significant vascularity (**Fig. 37**A, B, C, D). Fine-needle aspiration of the lymphangioma reveals straw-colored fluid and abundant

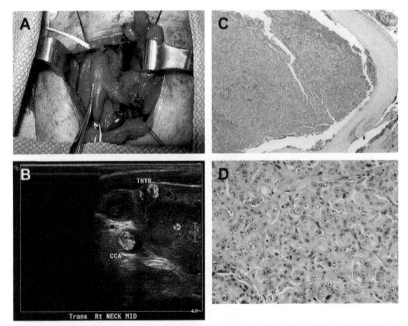

Fig. 35. (A) Occasionally a thyroid malignancy may extend into the middle thyroid vein and thereafter the internal jugular vein (IJV). (B) Transverse ultrasound image with Doppler demonstrates absence of IJV flow. (C) A cross section of the IJV demonstrates the thrombosis (hematoxylin and eosin, low power). (D) Histology of the thrombus demonstrates a poorly differentiated thyroid carcinoma.

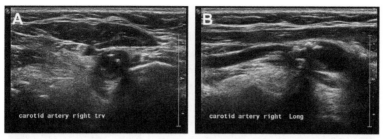

Fig. 36. (*A*, *B*) Atherosclerosis of the common carotid artery is indicated by calcification at the carotid bulb.

lymphocytes on cytology. A mass effect in the parotid may also represent a vascular anomaly. When a large vessel loop is noted on Doppler study, a more definitive vascular study such as CT angiogram may be warranted (**Fig. 38**A, B).

MISCELLANEOUS MASSES

A mass lesion in zone IIa may be a benign or malignant hyperplastic lymph node, second branchial cleft cyst, degenerated metastatic lymph node, or a neurogenic or vascular tumor. A carotid body tumor will demonstrate a mass at the bifurcation,

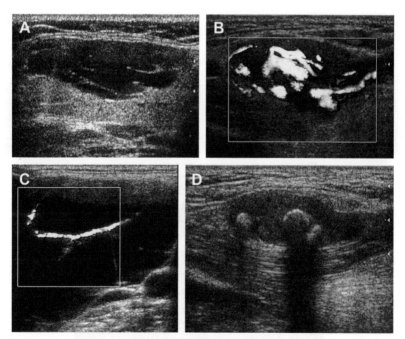

Fig. 37. (*A*) A hemangioma of the parotid gland demonstrates septations. (*B*) The parenchyma of the hemangioma demonstrates hypervascularity. (*C*) When vascularity is confined to the septations and absent in the parenchyma, a lymphangioma is suspected. (*D*) Calcifications are demonstrated in this hemangioma.

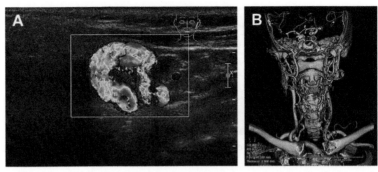

Fig. 38. (*A*) A parotid mass studied with Doppler demonstrates a large vessel loop. The ultrasound led to the diagnostic CT angiogram. (*B*) The vessel loop is from an anomalous internal carotid artery.

separation of the internal and external carotid arteries, and a hypervascular parenchyma (**Fig. 39**A, B). Doppler will demonstrate that the tumor vascularity arises from an independent vessel from the external carotid system, usually the ascending pharyngeal artery (see **Fig. 39**C). Neurogenic tumors arising from the sympathetic chain displace the carotid artery anteriorly and demonstrate a Horner syndrome clinically (**Fig. 40**A, B). A characteristic taper at the inferior end of the mass represents the

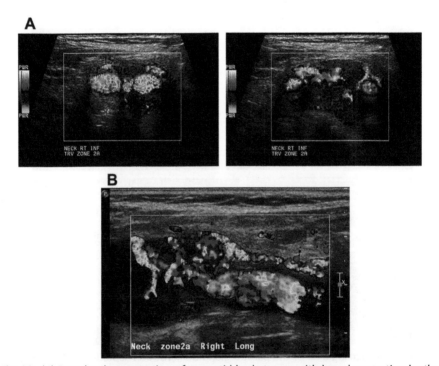

Fig. 39. (*A*) Doppler demonstration of a carotid body tumor with broad separation by the mass of the internal and external carotid arteries. (*B*) Sagittal Doppler view demonstrates the precise vascular supply to the carotid body tumor from the ascending pharyngeal artery.

A

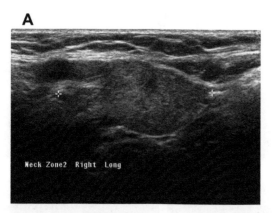

B

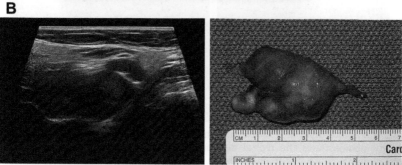

Fig. 40. (*A*) A neurofibroma arising from the sympathetic chain is demonstrated in zone IIa. (*B*) A comparison of the ultrasound image and actual pathology reveals the precision of ultrasound including the taper at the nerve exit from the tumor.

nerve of origin. A neurofibroma of the cervical plexus may also displace the carotid anteromedially, but there is no Horner syndrome. Again, a taper of the mass at the inferior end will indicate the association with the nerve of origin. Power Doppler confirms that the mass is not a vascular lesion.

THYROID LESIONS

Thyroid ultrasound has been covered in The Role of Ultrasound in Thyroid Disorders elsewhere in this issue. Here, some of the more common entities are described.

Hashimoto Thyroiditis

There are several distinct images that are demonstrative of thyroiditis (**Fig. 41**A, B). One of the key hallmarks of thyroiditis is the diffuse nature of the condition and bilateral and isthmus involvement. The thyroid is diffusely heterogeneous. One of the more typical images is a "Swiss cheese" pattern. There may be multiple pseudo nodule formations or hypoechoic streaking throughout the gland. The thyroid is relatively hypovascular. Riedel struma, a rare inflammatory condition, may resemble thyroiditis (**Fig. 42**A, B).

The rigid texture and lack of cellularity on fine-needle aspiration cytology may require core biopsy for definitive diagnosis (see **Fig. 42**C).

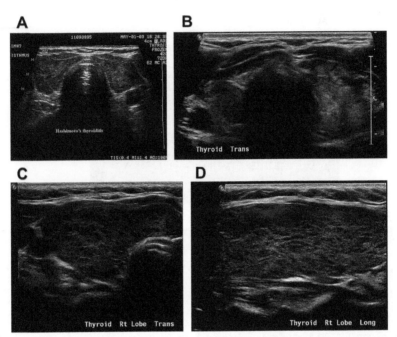

Fig. 41. Hashimoto thyroiditis may demonstrate a variety of patterns. (*A*) One example of thyroiditis demonstrates the typical disappearance of thyroid parenchyma. (*B*) Another form may demonstrate thyromegaly and hypoechoic streaking and pseudonodule formation. (*C, D*) A "Swiss cheese" pattern is frequently noted on ultrasound.

Graves Disease

The thyroid may be significantly enlarged or even relatively normal in size. Power Doppler always demonstrates diffuse hypervascularity (**Fig. 43**).

Multinodular Goiter

There are many sonographic variations of nodular goiter. Nodules may be hypoechoic, hyperechoic, or anechoic and vary in size and position. Coarse calcifications are common. Occasionally, the inferior extent of the thyroid cannot be determined on ultrasound, requiring CT scan to determine the degree of substernal extension. The isthmus must be carefully assessed, as it is easy to forget that it can harbor large nodules or significant pathology. One of the most difficult concepts in assessment of multinodular goiter is to determine which nodules to biopsy. The "dominant" nodule is the largest of multiple nodules and traditionally the one most likely to be biopsied; however, there are other nodule characteristics that may require biopsy. Irregularity, infiltration of strap muscles, hypervascularity, and microcalcifications are some of the features that demand biopsy.

Single Nodule

A single anechoic nodule that has a distinct hypoechoic halo and is hypovascular often represents a follicular lesion. A single nodule that reveals microcalcifications, irregular margins, and hypervascularity on Doppler is suspicious for papillary carcinoma (**Fig. 44**A, B, C, D). Medullary carcinoma can demonstrate microcalcifications.

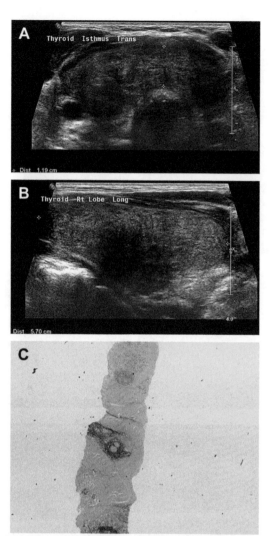

Fig. 42. (*A, B*) A rare inflammatory condition, Riedel struma, demonstrates diffuse fibrosis on both sagittal and transverse views. (*C*) A core biopsy is frequently required as the fibrosis does not demonstrate on fine-needle aspiration (H & E, low power).

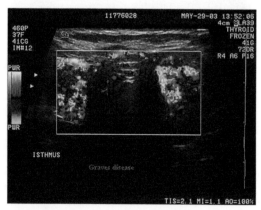

Fig. 43. In contrast to an enlarged thyroid gland with Hashimoto thyroiditis, Graves disease demonstrates diffuse hypervascularity with power Doppler.

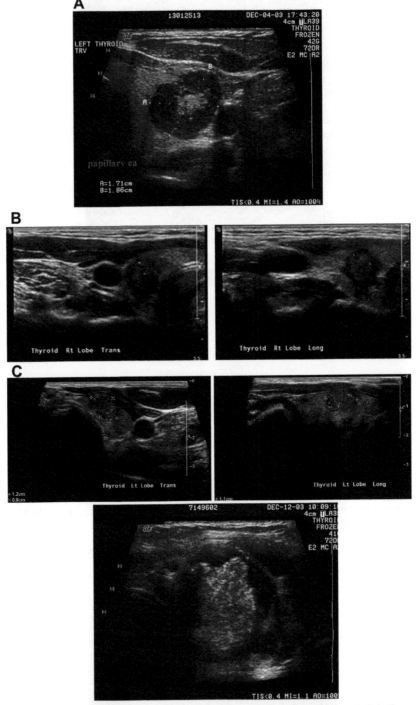

Fig. 44. Papillary carcinoma has several identifying features on ultrasound. (*A*) The mass may be cystic. (*B*) The margins may be irregular. (*C*) Diffuse microcalcifications are common. (*D*) Power Doppler often demonstrates that the mass is hypervascular.

D

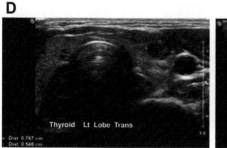
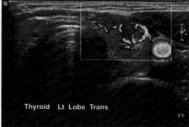

Fig. 44. (*continued*)

Anechoic nodules may be either adenomatous or cysts. Of course, obvious associated suspicious adenopathy should raise the possible question of a relationship to the single thyroid nodule. Thyroid lymphoma is a more diffuse process and replaces the entire lobe or full gland (**Fig. 45**A, B).

PARATHYROID LESIONS

The normal parathyroid glands are below the resolution ability of ultrasound. Primary hyperparathyroidism is most commonly the result of a single adenoma. The parathyroid adenoma is hypoechoic and nearly anechoic in architecture. It is also classically located. The inferior adenoma is at or near the inferior pole of the thyroid and immediately adjacent to the thyroid capsule (**Fig. 46**). The superior parathyroid adenoma is at or craniad to the midpoint of the thyroid gland (**Fig. 47**). When ectopic, the superior parathyroid may even be inferior to the position of the normal inferior parathyroid gland and may locate to the area adjacent to the esophagus (**Fig. 48**). Frequently the inferior parathyroid adenoma is in the thymic tongue and is still identifiable with ultrasound (**Fig. 49**).

Diffuse hyperplasia is suspected when 2 or more enlarged parathyroids are identified (**Fig. 50**A, B). Occasionally, a parathyroid adenoma is difficult to distinguish from a hyperplastic lymph node. One of the key differentiating features is the vascular pattern of the adenoma on Doppler. A discrete vessel (parathyroid artery, a branch of the inferior thyroid artery) is identified anterior to the adenoma and ends bluntly in the parenchyma of the mass (**Fig. 51**A, B, C, D). In contrast, the vascular pattern of a lymph node classically arborizes within the node and a dominant adjacent vessel is less likely (**Fig. 52**). When a parathyroid adenoma cannot be identified in any cardinal

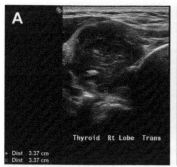
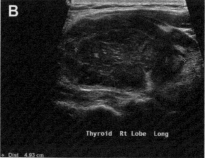

Fig. 45. (*A, B*) A thyroid lymphoma diffusely replaces the normal thyroid parenchyma.

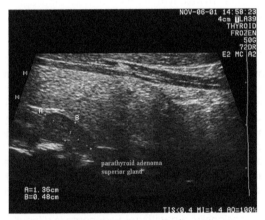

Fig. 46. An inferior parathyroid adenoma is demonstrated in an extracapsular location with hypoechoic architecture and a typical ovoid configuration.

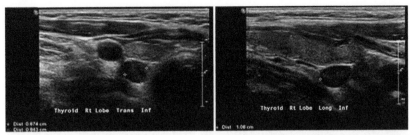

Fig. 47. A superior parathyroid adenoma in its cardinal position.

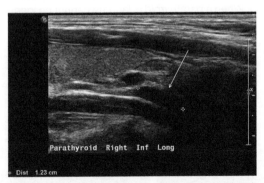

Fig. 48. An ectopic and hypertrophied superior parathyroid gland is demonstrated on this sagittal view of a patient with MEN I. The arrow points to the superior adenoma adjacent to the more typically located enlarged inferior parathyroid gland.

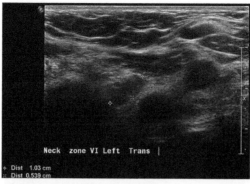

Fig. 49. Inferior parathyroid gland within the thymus.

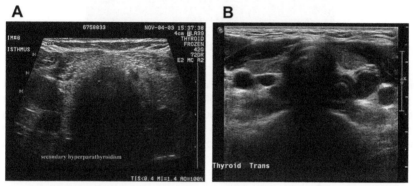

Fig. 50. (*A*) Marked enlargement of all parathyroid glands is noted in secondary hyperparathyroidism from renal disease. (*B*) Three enlarged parathyroid glands are demonstrated in this single transverse plane in a patient with MEN I.

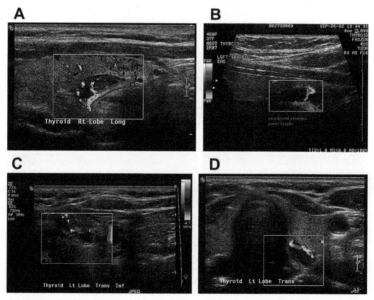

Fig. 51. (*A, B, C, D*) The vascular pattern of a typical parathyroid adenoma demonstrates a well-defined parathyroid artery that ends bluntly in the adenoma parenchyma. Four separate cases are demonstrated.

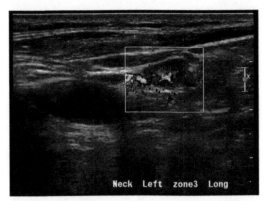

Fig. 52. In contrast to the vascular pattern of a parathyroid adenoma, a hyperplastic lymph node demonstrates an arborizing pattern within the node.

position, an ectopic position is likely. The thymus, carotid sheath and area adjacent to the pyriform sinus are consistent regions of investigation. The intrathyroidal adenoma can be identified on preoperative ultrasound (**Fig. 53**A). Again, a dominant single vessel can usually be noted entering the intrathyroidal adenoma, which otherwise cannot be distinguished sonographically from a simple thyroid adenoma. Occasionally

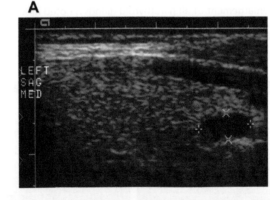

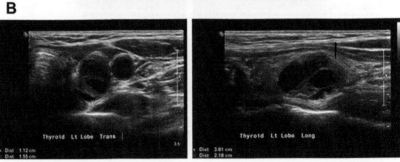

Fig. 53. (A) An intrathyroidal parathyroid adenoma is completely surrounded by normal thyroid parenchyma. (B) The intrathyroidal parathyroid adenoma may demonstrate cystic degeneration and require parathyroid hormone assessment of its fluid for confirmation.

a large intrathyroidal adenoma becomes cystic and may be misinterpreted as a complex thyroid nodule or cyst (see **Fig. 53**B). In this circumstance, a fine-needle aspiration for a parathyroid hormone will determine the true nature of the lesion in question.

TEMPOROMANDIBULAR JOINT AND MANDIBLE

Temporomandibular joint arthritis or other deficits may be identified on ultrasound. Occasionally, a joint effusion is noted when one side is compared with the normal asymptomatic joint. A cyst in the parotid gland adjacent to the mandibular condyle may be of synovial origin from the joint. An example of this circumstance demonstrates the precise connection of the cyst to the joint, which was not determined on any other imaging modality including fine-cut CT scan (**Fig. 54**A, B, C).

ULTRASOUND BY THE OTOLARYNGOLOGIST FOR DIAGNOSIS

These are but a few examples of the comprehensive application of ultrasound to the diagnosis and management of head and neck lesions. In the hands of the clinician, real-time examination of relevant anatomy adds immeasurably to the understanding

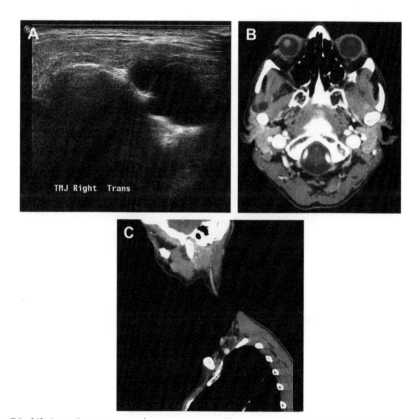

Fig. 54. (*A*) A cystic mass near the temporomandibular joint may not be of parotid origin. This ultrasound demonstrates the connection between this cyst and the joint, which confirms the diagnosis of a synovial cyst. (*B, C*) CT scans do not adequately demonstrate this relationship.

of the condition at hand. This procedure allows more efficient and precise management of thyroid nodules at selected intervals because the same examiner is performing the assessment each time. Any lesion of interest is amenable to fine-needle aspiration cytology, which often can be performed during the same visit. This process is more efficient for patients and will be cost effective. Most importantly, when ultrasound becomes common practice for clinicians, new previously undetermined applications of this modality will evolve and add to the body of diagnostic knowledge.

REFERENCES

1. Ahuja A, Evans R. Practical head and neck ultrasound. London: Greenwich Medical Media Limited; 2000.
2. Liao LJ, Wang CT, Young YH, et al. Real-time and computerized sonographic scoring system for predicting malignant cervical lymphadenopathy. Head and Neck 2010;32:594–8.

The Expanding Utility of Office-Based Ultrasound for the Head and Neck Surgeon

Jeffrey M. Bumpous, MD[a], Gregory W. Randolph, MD[b],*

KEYWORDS

• Ultrasound • Head and neck surgery • Office-based ultrasound

ULTRASOUND FOR THE HEAD AND NECK SURGEON

Ultrasound has increasingly moved from being a modality confined to the radiology department to an active diagnostic and therapeutic aid available to the head and neck at the point of patient care.[1] Ultrasound as a modality offers several advantages, including small size, low cost of instrumentation, steadily improving resolution, and lack of ionizing radiation and can readily be incorporated into a surgeon's algorithm for determining risk of malignancy in lymph nodes and thyroid nodules.[1,2] The clinical application of ultrasound for head and neck surgeons continues to evolve with increasing levels of information derived from the technology, increasing numbers of practitioners becoming familiar with ultrasound, and a rapidly expanding volume of literature. A PubMed search from January 1, 2000, to January 1, 2010, revealed 1800 articles regarding the use of ultrasound in the head and neck (almost 5 articles per day).

The use of ultrasound has become increasingly sophisticated with 2-D imaging as well as Doppler flow, which help characterize vascular patterns, in particular for hyperechoic foci within the thyroid gland to distinguish vessels from cystic masses. Addition of advanced ultrasound techniques, such as elastography, increases ultrasound specificity in detecting thyroid malignancy.[2,3] Increasingly, there are ultrasound-related courses and didactic training for practicing physicians. Formal ultrasonography head and neck curricula exist, for example, in the postgraduate medical education head and neck ultrasound course of the American College of Surgeons.

[a] Department of Surgery, University of Louisville, University Surgical Associates, PSC, 401 East Chestnut Street, Suite 710, Louisville, KY 40202, USA
[b] Massachusetts Eye and Ear Infirmary, 243 Charles Street, Boston, MA 02114, USA
* Corresponding author.
E-mail address: Gregory_Randolph@meei.harvard.edu

Otolaryngol Clin N Am 43 (2010) 1203–1208
doi:10.1016/j.otc.2010.08.009
0030-6665/10/$ – see front matter © 2010 Published by Elsevier Inc.

oto.theclinics.com

In order to optimize safety and accuracy of ultrasonography in an otolaryngology practice, systematic application of the modality with full knowledge of the strengths and weaknesses of the modality must be appreciated.[2]

BASICS OF ULTRASOUND TECHNOLOGY FOR THE OFFICE

There are many clinical ultrasound systems available for clinical use in the office and at the bedside. Small size, portability, and affordability of this equipment have made it more available and attractive to clinical practice. System requirements can be viewed as basic and advanced. More advanced components may require increasing levels of training for accurate use. **Table 1** lists basic and advanced requirements for office-based ultrasound systems.[1]

EVALUATION TECHNIQUE: AN ANATOMIC APPROACH

Development of a systematic approach to performing head and neck office-based ultrasonography is paramount in order to adequately assess pathology and not miss potentially important clinical findings. **Fig. 1** outlines a systematic approach to head and neck ultrasonography and represents only one organizational scheme. The examination should include the central or visceral compartment of the neck in both longitudinal and transverse planes. Within the central compartment, attention is directed at the endocrine organs (thyroid and parathyroid), trachea, esophagus, and paratracheal and prelaryngeal and pretracheal lymph nodes. In the postoperative neck of well-differentiated thyroid cancer patients, accurate reporting of size, location, and character of lymph nodes is important to assess for disease progression. The lateral neck must also be evaluated in patients with thyroid cancer; failure to do so results in poor sensitivity of the examination in detection of lymphadenopathy.[1,2,4]

THYROID ULTRASOUND

With respect to the thyroid gland, the dimensions of both lobes and the isthmus should be assessed and recorded, which requires assessment in the longitudinal and transverse planes. Size, location, and echo characteristics should also be recorded. Vascular patterns surrounding nodules from Doppler flow may provide etiologic clues.[1,2,4] Any calcifications should be noted and preferably recorded as static images. A pattern of microcalcification in a nodule significantly increases the risk that the nodule may be malignant. In the multinodular thyroid gland, ultrasound is

Table 1		
Basic and advanced requirements for head and neck office-based ultrasound systems		
Component	**Basic**	**Advanced**
Ultrasound machine	1. High frequency (7.5–14 MHz) 2. A and B modes 3. Color-coded duplex (enhances differentiation of cystic areas and vascularity)	1. 3-D ultrasound 2. Elastography
Education	1. American College of Surgeons course 2. American Academy of Otolaryngology	1. Radiological Society of North America 2. American Association of Clinical Endocrinologists

Data from Lyshchilk AH. Thyroid gland tumor. Radiology 2005;237(1):202–11.

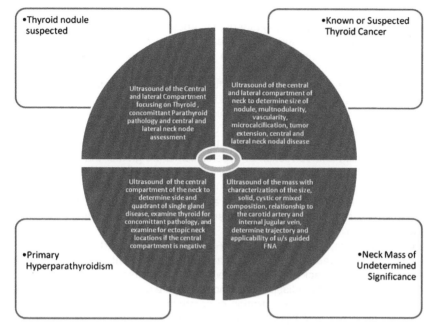

Fig. 1. Systematic application of head and neck ultrasonography.

particularly helpful in recognizing areas within the gland that are at higher risk of malignancy, such as nodules greater than 1 cm and those possessing hypervascularity and microcalcification.[2] Limitations of ultrasound in thyroid assessment include assessment of substernal extent of the gland, predicting airway invasion, distinguishing coexistent lymph node from parathyroid pathology, and lack of definitive pathologic characteristics in the context of a multinodular gland.[1,4] **Table 2** lists common characteristics of thyroid malignancy on ultrasound.

PARATHYROID ULTRASOUND

The parathyroid glands in the normal state are difficult to precisely identify in many state-of-the-art imaging modalities, including ultrasound.[5] In the case of primary

| Table 2 |
Ultrasound characteristics of thyroid malignancy
Size >1 cm and solid
Microcalcification
Central blood flow pattern
Strain index >4 on offline elastograms (96% specificity, 82% sensitivity)
Margin regularity score (88% specificity, 36% sensitivity)
Tumor area ratio >1 (92% specificity, 46% sensitivity)

Data from Welkoborsky HJ. Ultrasound usage in the head and neck surgeon's office. Curr Opin Otolaryngol Head Neck Surg 2009;17(2):116–21; and Lyshchilk AH. Thyroid gland tumor. Radiology 2005;237(1):202–11.

hyperparathyroidism, however, ultrasound of the central compartment may be diagnostic of single-gland disease (adenoma). Anatomic relationships to the trachea, larynx, esophagus, thyroid, and carotid sheath contents may allow for identification of diseased parathyroid glands and provide information regarding side and upper or lower position.

In cases of positive nuclear medicine studies, such as technetium 99m sestamibi scan, ultrasound may provide more refined information regarding anatomic location of the adenoma than nuclear medicine study alone.[5,6] In cases of suspicious yet equivocal nuclear medicine evaluations, office-based ultrasonography can provide concordance. If the two examinations are concordant, the correlations with successful unilateral surgical exploration and correction of hypercalcemia are greater than 95%.[7] Several studies have demonstrated success in localizing single-gland disease in cases of negative nuclear medicine studies, arguably making this modality the most useful modality in parathyroid localization; this in part may be a result of high-resolution ultrasound; when read by an experienced ultrasonographer, it may allow identification parathyroid adenomas as small as 0.5 cm.[5]

In clinical practice, localization of single- versus multiple-gland disease may often be aided by office ultrasound and nuclear medicine assessment. Additionally, ectopic locations in the lateral neck and submandibular triangle are readily accessible for ultrasound examination, but mediastinal ectopic glands are not often identified with ultrasound. Critics of ultrasound localization of parathyroid adenoma suggest that there are limitations in resolution (without high-resolution scanners), potential confusion with paratracheal lymph nodes, and difficulty in imaging below the clavicles.[5–7]

NECK LYMPHATICS ULTRASOUND

Examination of the lymphatics of the neck by office-based ultrasound is pertinent in evaluation of myriad pathologies, including upper aerodigestive, thyroid, and parathyroid malignancy as well as benign lymphadenopathy and other neck masses. Size greater than 1 cm, clustering of nodes, rounding of shape, peripheral vascularity, cystic (hyperechoic) change, microcalcification, and loss of a distinguishable fatty hilum on ultrasound are all characteristics of malignancy within cervical nodes.[8] Ultrasound provides an objective means of documenting lymph node size, location, and characteristics and can, therefore, be useful in following equivocal areas for progression in size. In particular, ultrasound is useful for post-thyroidectomy follow-up of patients with an established diagnosis of well-differentiated thyroid carcinoma. Early baseline examination (with or without needle biopsy) and subsequent follow-up examinations provide a context for evaluating both central compartment and lateral lymph nodes for growth.[2,8–10] Preoperative ultrasound evaluation of the lateral neck in high-risk patients with well-differentiated thyroid cancer may allow for more appropriate inclusion or exclusion of lateral compartment lymphadenectomy.[10] In cases of elevated thyroglobulin in post-thyroidectomy, well-differentiated thyroid carcinomas, ultrasound can provide a low-cost and accurate means of reassessing the thyroid bed and cervical nodal basin. Ultrasound represents an effective and low-cost modality that may supplement or even obviate iodine scan or PET scan in situations where thyroglobulin is elevated.[11] Additionally, ultrasound provides superior opportunity for needle-based biopsy than nuclear medicine studies; is less expensive than other image-guided biopsy modalities, such as CT and MRI; and may also be useful in directed needle-based interventions in poorly accessible or nonpalpable areas (ie, alcohol injection of small metastatic nodes).[2,8,9,11]

OFFICE-BASED HEAD AND NECK ULTRASOUND BIOPSY

Ultrasound-guided needle aspiration biopsy is a well-accepted modality for biopsy of head and neck masses from salivary to endocrine to lymphatic tissues.[2] Ultrasound-guided needle biopsy of head and neck masses should be preceded by adequate history, physical examination, and diagnostic ultrasound of the pathology in question as well as surrounding head and neck structural relationships.[1,2,4,9] Optimal diagnostic success occurs when there is communication between the clinician and pathologist to make certain there is adequate sample retrieved and that the sample is processed appropriately. Office-based ultrasound-guided biopsy of thyroid, parathyroid, lymphatic and other neck masses allows for more prompt diagnosis. The technical process of ultrasound-guided needle biopsy in the head and neck is beyond the scope of this article, but the techniques are increasingly emphasized in well-vetted courses that are available to head and neck surgeons.

THERAPEUTIC APPLICATIONS OF HEAD AND NECK ULTRASOUND

Ultrasound in many areas has become an accepted modality for guidance of therapeutic interventions ranging from alcohol injections to radiofrequency ablation.[11] The literature and experience with ultrasound-guided therapeutic interventions in the head and neck are more limited and without data from large multi-institutional clinical trials. Ultrasound-guided alcohol injection has been reported in ablation of primary thyroid lesions as well as lymph nodes bearing evidence of papillary thyroid carcinoma. Proposed use in parathyroid adenomas is controversial.[11] The lack of a thick capsule in parathyroid adenomas may allow for diffusion of alcohol injections and result in collateral tissue damage, in particular the inferior (recurrent) or superior laryngeal nerves. Cases of recurrent laryngeal nerve paralysis after alcohol injection have been reported.[12,13] Radiofrequency ablation is a modality that is commonly used for areas, such as hepatic lesions. Ultrasound-guided radiofrequency ablation requires additional expertise in understanding microwave technology and its tissue effects. Radiofrequency ablation has been used successfully in the treatment of head and neck lesions and has been reported as an alternative to surgery in selected patients.[14] Pain, hematoma, and voice change are among the reported complications of ultrasound radiofrequency ablation of thyroid lesions.[15,16] Coupled with ultrasound, appropriate training in the interpretation of imaging endpoints, radiofrequency ablation may provide an area of further potential therapeutic intervention for head and neck surgeons.

INTEGRATION OF OFFICE-BASED ULTRASONOGRAPHY

Office-based ultrasonography is increasingly being integrated into the practice of otolaryngology–head and neck surgery. Use of a systematic anatomic-based approach provides increased diagnostic information and opportunities for more refined disease management in thyroid, parathyroid, and upper aerodigestive tract masses and malignancies. Adequate training for appropriate technical execution and clinical interpretation of head and neck disease findings on ultrasound are increasingly available in postgraduate medical education and continuing medical education formats. Unique imaging characteristics, low cost, correlation with clinical examination, and pre-existing anatomic and clinical knowledge of head and neck disease processes make the inclusion of office-based ultrasound for head and neck surgeons an attractive prospect. Ultrasound complements a physical examination in the postoperative or postirradiated neck. In addition to the general diagnostic information of ultrasound, guided biopsy provides an opportunity for precision in the office for fine-needle aspiration of masses that are not readily palpable. Although not well established (due to lack of large-scale clinical trial data), ultrasound-guided therapeutic intervention is an additional area that head and neck surgeons should continue to have awareness of as it enters practice. Ultrasound-based interventions will need critical evaluation for safety and efficacy.

REFERENCES

1. Charous SJ. An overview of office-based ultrasonography: new versions. Otolaryngol Head Neck Surg 2004;131(6):1001–3.
2. Welkoborsky HJ. Ultrasound usage in the head and neck surgeon's office. Curr Opin Otolaryngol Head Neck Surg 2009;17(2):116–21.
3. Lyshchilk AH. Thyroid gland tumor. Radiology 2005;237(1):202–11.
4. Slough CM. Workup of well-differentiated thyroid carcinoma. Cancer Control 2006;13(2):99–105.
5. Gurney TA. Otolaryngologist-head and neck surgeon performed ultrasonography for identification for parathyroid adenoma localization. Laryngoscope 2008;118: 243–6.
6. Bumpous JM. Surgical and calcium outcomes in 427 patients treated prospectively in an image guided and intraoperative PTH supplemented protocol for primary hyperparathyroidism. Laryngoscope 2009;119:300–6.
7. Lal G. Primary hyperparathyroidism: controversies in surgical management. Trends Endocrinol Metab 2003;14(9):417–22.
8. Gritzman NH. Sonography of soft tissue masses of the neck. J Clin Ultrasound 2002;30:356–73.
9. Ahuja A. Sonographic evaluation of cervical lymph nodes. American Journal of Roentgenology 2004;184:1691–9.
10. Davidson HC. Papillary thyroid cancer: controversies in the management of neck metastasis. Laryngoscope 2008;118:2161–5.
11. Johnson NA. Postoperative surveillance of differentiated thyroid carcinoma: rational, techniques and controversies. Radiology 2008;249(2):429–44.
12. Maus PS. Complications of ultrasound guided percutaneous ethanol injection therapy of the thyroid and parathyroid glands. Ultraschall Med 2005;26(2):142–5.
13. Brzac H. Ultrasonography-guided therapeutic procedures in the neck. Acta Med Croatica 2009;63(3):21–7.
14. Baek J. Benign predominantly solid thyroid nodules: prospective study of efficacy of sonographically guided radiofrequency ablation versus control condition. (AJR) Am J Roengtenol 2010;194:1137–42.
15. Jeong WB. Radiofrequency ablation of benign thyroid nodules: safety and imaging follow-up in 236 patients. Eur Radiol 2008;18(6):1244–50.
16. Monchik JM. Radiofrequency ablation and percutaneous ethanol injection treatment for recurrent local and distant well-differentiated thyroid carcinoma. Ann Surg 2006;244(2):296–304.

Role of Ultrasound in Thyroid Disorders

Gerald T. Kangelaris, MD[a], Theresa B. Kim, MD[a,b],
Lisa A. Orloff, MD[c],*

KEYWORDS

- Thyroid ultrasound • Thyroid cancer • Thyroid nodule
- Thyroid FNA • Ultrasonography

HISTORICAL PERSPECTIVE OF THYROID ULTRASOUND

Thyroid ultrasonography commands a central role in the evaluation, diagnosis, and treatment of thyroid disorders. Ultrasound has been the standard for imaging of the thyroid gland for many years and is the first-line recommended imaging modality for thyroid nodules.[1,2] Its use in thyroid disorders is widely accepted and the benefits and indications for its use continue to expand. Thyroid ultrasonography has traditionally been under the purview of radiology departments, but in the past decade has been adopted by surgeons and endocrinologists in the office-based setting for evaluation and management of patients with thyroid and other head and neck disorders. Its versatility, speed, safety profile, ability to offer dynamic real-time images, and low cost compared with other radiologic modalities have all contributed to its popularity.

The initial uses of thyroid ultrasonography came at a time when palpable thyroid nodules were surgically excised to establish a pathologic diagnosis. In the late 1960s, ultrasound was used to differentiate between solid and cystic nodules and to measure and track nodule size.[3] Using conventional ultrasonography without the benefit of gray-scale images, clinicians were able to differentiate cysts from cystic degeneration in an adenoma, solid tumors from multinodular goiter, and to detect the presence of thyroiditis with greater than 90% accuracy.[4,5] However, the differentiation of benign versus malignant lesions remained problematic, and in the following decade, investigators began studying whether newer ultrasound technology could

Funding support: the authors have no financial support to disclose.
[a] Department of Otolaryngology – Head & Neck Surgery, University of California, San Francisco, 2380 Sutter Street, 1st Floor, Campus Box 0342, San Francisco, CA 94115, USA
[b] Department of Otolaryngology, Pediatric Otolaryngology, 1 Children's Place, Suite 3S35, St Louis, MO 63110, USA
[c] Department of Otolaryngology–Head & Neck Surgery, University of California, San Francisco, 2380 Sutter Street, 2nd Floor, San Francisco, CA 94115, USA
* Corresponding author.
E-mail address: lorloff@ohns.ucsf.edu

help improve surgical and medical decision making by identifying malignant features of thyroid lesions.[6]

In the past 40 years, the role of thyroid ultrasonography has continued to expand and it is currently recommended in the evaluation of all palpable nodules by the American Thyroid Association (ATA), the American Association of Clinical Endocrinologists (AACE), and the Associazione Medici Endocrinologi (AME).[1,2] The thyroid gland is well suited to ultrasound evaluation in part because of the superficial position and easy accessibility of the gland, its distinctive echotexture, and the ability to gain greater anatomic detail than with computed tomography, magnetic resonance imaging, or radionuclide studies. **Table 1** lists some of the goals of and indications for thyroid ultrasonography.

This article reviews the relevant uses of and indications for ultrasound in various thyroid diseases, with particular attention to thyroid nodules and cancer. The characteristic ultrasound features of these diseases are described. The associated literature and societal guidelines are discussed.

ROLE OF ULTRASOUND IN THE INITIAL EVALUATION OF THE THYROID NODULE

The ATA and AACE/AME recommend thyroid ultrasound for all patients with suspected thyroid nodules,[1,2] including patients with palpable abnormalities, nodular goiter, and thyroid lesions found incidentally on other imaging modalities. Routine

Table 1
Thyroid ultrasonography goals and indications

To better assess palpable thyroid nodules	To facilitate FNA biopsy of a nodule
To determine whether nodularity is present in the patient with an equivocal or difficult physical examination	To assess the remainder of the thyroid gland in the patient with a palpable thyroid nodule
To determine whether characteristics associated with malignancy are present	To screen for thyroid lesions in patients who have been exposed to radiation
To screen for thyroid lesions in patients with other diseases in the neck, such as hyperparathyroidism, who are undergoing treatment planning	To objectively monitor nodules, goiters, or lymph nodes in patients undergoing treatment or observation of thyroid disease
To assess the thyroid and the extrathyroid neck in the patient with thyroid cancer before treatment	To monitor treated patients with thyroid cancer for early evidence of recurrence in the thyroid bed and cervical lymph nodes
To identify thyroid features associated with diseases including thyroiditis and Graves disease	To facilitate therapeutic procedures such as sclerotherapy or laser ablation of thyroid nodules
To help teach regional anatomy and the art of thyroid palpation	To detect undescended thyroid or thyroid agenesis
To monitor fetal thyroid development in utero	To assess the size and location of the neonatal thyroid
To detect goiter as a sign of iodine deficiency	To refine management of patients on therapy such as antithyroid medications
To screen family members of patients with familial forms of thyroid cancer	

Data from Morris LF, Ragavendra N, Yeh MW. Evidence-based assessment of the role of ultrasonography in the management of benign thyroid nodules. World J Surg 2008;32:1253–63; Orloff LA. Head and neck ultrasonography. Plural Publishing; 2008.

screening thyroid ultrasound is not recommended for the general population because of the high incidence of thyroid nodules. An autopsy study of 821 consecutive patients with clinically normal thyroid glands showed that 50% of patients had at least one thyroid nodule and 36% had nodules greater than 2 cm in size.[7] Palpable thyroid nodules occur in up to 7% of the general adult population, and the incidence of non-palpable thyroid nodules visible by ultrasound is up to 10 times greater (ie, 70%).[8–10]

Ultrasound evaluation of thyroid nodules in at-risk patients can help confirm the presence of a nodule; objectively characterize the size, location, and appearance of the nodule; evaluate for benign or suspicious features; and evaluate for the presence of other thyroid nodules or cervical lymphadenopathy.[1] Although certain ultrasound characteristics of thyroid nodules are associated with malignancy, fine-needle aspiration (FNA) remains the gold standard for diagnosis. FNA has until recently been recommended for cytologic evaluation of all thyroid nodules greater than 1 cm in diameter or nodules less than 1 cm that exhibit suspicious features.[1,2] The 2009 Revised ATA Guidelines for Management of Thyroid Nodules and Differentiated Thyroid Cancer also include recommendations for FNA of certain thyroid lesions based on ultrasound criteria. These criteria include mixed solid and cystic nodules 1.5 to 2 cm or greater in diameter with any suspicious ultrasound characteristics and predominantly spongi-form nodules 2 cm or greater in diameter.[1] Although considered the gold standard, the diagnostic role of FNA is limited by an overall 3% to 5% false-negative rate and a 10% nondiagnostic rate.[11]

The use of ultrasound guidance improves the sensitivity, specificity, and accuracy of FNA compared with palpation-guided FNA in certain populations.[12–15] Ultrasound-guided FNA seems to be most valuable in patients with nonpalpable nodules, small palpable nodules, multiple nodules, partially cystic nodules, or concomitant glandular disease. It is also beneficial for sampling specific areas of a nodule, such as from the solid part of a mixed solid-cystic nodule. Compared with palpation-guided FNA, the-use of ultrasound guidance decreased the rate of inadequate samples in palpable nodules 2 cm or smaller from 39% to 23%.[14] Cesur and colleagues[12] found the rates of inadequate FNA samples to be significantly improved in palpable nodules 1.0 to 1.5 cm using ultrasound- versus palpation-guided FNA (37.6% vs 24.4%, $P = .009$), but not for palpable nodules 1.6 cm or larger. Currently, the ATA recommends ultra-sound-guided FNA for nodules that are nonpalpable, predominately cystic, or located posteriorly in the thyroid lobe, and when repeating FNA for a nodule with an initial non-diagnostic cytology result.[1]

ULTRASOUND CHARACTERISTICS OF THYROID NODULES

Many investigators have identified ultrasound characteristics of malignant thyroid nodules (**Table 2**). Although these ultrasound characteristics offer high sensitivity, no single criterion offers sufficient specificity to differentiate benign from malignant lesions.[16] However, when taken together, specificity improves. One prospective, observational study compared ultrasound and FNA results with surgical disease conditions in 349 patients and found that performing FNA on nodules with one of 3 ultrasound criteria (microcalcifications, blurred margins, or hypoechoic pattern) missed only 2% of cancers.[17] Kim and colleagues[18] prospectively analyzed 155 inci-dentally discovered, nonpalpable, solid thyroid nodules and found a mean number of 2.6 suspicious findings per malignant nodule and an overall sensitivity and specificity of 94% and 66%, respectively.

The next sections discuss ultrasound features of thyroid nodules and their ability to suggest benign versus malignant lesions.

Table 2 Ultrasound features associated with malignancy	
Margins	Blurred, ill-defined
Halo/rim	Absent
Shape	Irregular, spherical, tall
Echo structure	Solid
Echogenicity	Hypoechoic
Calcifications	Microcalcifications, internal
Vascular pattern	Intranodular, hypervascular
Elastography	Decreased elasticity

Data from Morris LF, Ragavendra N, Yeh MW. Evidence-based assessment of the role of ultrasonography in the management of benign thyroid nodules. World J Surg 2008;32:1253–63.

NODULE SIZE

Nodule size has not been found to be significantly predictive of malignancy. The risk of malignancy for palpable thyroid nodules is approximately 10% and several studies suggest a similar incidence of malignancy in nodules smaller than 1 cm.[19–21] Thyroid cancers less than 1 cm in size have been shown to behave clinically similar to larger cancers, and therefore these lesions should be followed with periodic ultrasound surveillance with the option for further evaluation with FNA if growth or suspicious features are observed.[22] The ATA recommends FNA biopsy of subcentimeter nodules if there is a high risk of malignancy (family history of thyroid cancer, history of external beam or ionizing radiation, history of thyroid cancer, or fluorodeoxyglucose-avid thyroid nodules on positron emission tomography) or if there is suspicious concomitant lymphadenopathy, in which case FNA of the lymph node should be performed.[1]

LESION MARGINS AND HALO/RIM

Benign lesions are often associated with a hypoechoic circumferential halo (**Fig. 1**), believed to represent a capsule and compressed thyroid tissue.[23] Neoplasms may display a partial or absent halo,[24] and its presence or absence has been found to be suggestive but not diagnostic.[24,25] Blurred or ill-defined margins have been associated with increased risk of malignancy.[17,24,25] The mobility of the nodule with respect to surrounding structures should be assessed, as fixation suggests malignant invasion of the surrounding tissue.

NODULE SHAPE

Nodule shape has been implicated as having prognostic significance. One retrospective analysis found nodules with a more spherical shape had a higher incidence of malignancy.[23] In contrast, another study found that nodules that are more tall than wide are more likely to harbor cancer.[18] Irregular shape has also been implicated in malignancy.[24]

ECHO STRUCTURE

Many thyroid nodules are cystic or have cystic components, such as cystic degeneration of a follicular adenoma (**Fig. 2**) or in the setting of multinodular goiter. Malignancy has been more closely associated with solid nodules compared with cystic or mixed nodules, with one study finding 121 of 148 (81.8%) histopathologically malignant

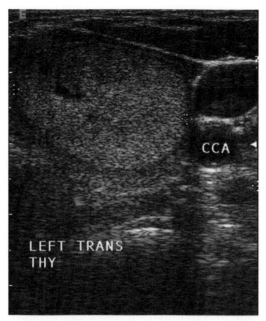

Fig. 1. Thin hypoechoic circumferential halo surrounding a benign thyroid nodule.

nodules to be solid.[17,24] Purely cystic nodules are unlikely to be malignant,[26] as are those with a spongiform appearance (**Fig. 3**), defined as an aggregation of multiple microcystic components in more than 50% of the nodal volume.[27,28]

ECHOGENICITY

The echogenicity of a thyroid nodule should be compared with that of surrounding thyroid tissue. Most benign adenomas or adenomatous nodules are slightly hypoechoic when compared with normal thyroid tissue (**Fig. 4**), whereas malignant nodules are frequently markedly hypoechoic (**Fig. 5**).[18,24] In a prospective, observational study of 349 surgically excised thyroid nodules, Cappelli and colleagues[17] found a 3.8 odds ratio of malignancy in solid hypoechoic nodules.

CALCIFICATIONS

The presence of calcifications has variable significance. Peripheral calcification, also referred to as eggshell calcification, is typically considered a benign feature, representing previous hemorrhage and degenerative change (**Fig. 6**). However, coarse calcifications can be seen in malignant nodules, as can microcalcifications, which are strongly associated with an increased risk of malignancy.[17] A total of 45% to 60% of malignant nodules show microcalcifications, as opposed to 7% to 14% of benign nodules.[18,29] Approximately 60% of patients with microcalcifications were found to have malignant disease.[30] The presence of microcalcifications in malignant nodules is often attributed to psammoma bodies in papillary thyroid carcinoma (PTC) (**Fig. 7**) and is frequently seen in medullary thyroid carcinoma (MTC). Although suggestive of malignancy, the overall specificity of microcalcifications for thyroid carcinoma has been reported to range from 71% to 94%, with a sensitivity of 35%

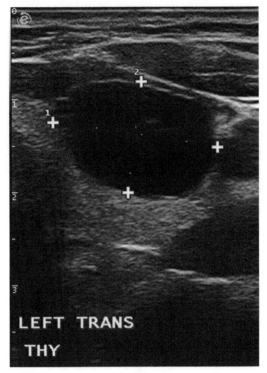

Fig. 2. Cystic degeneration of a benign thyroid nodule.

to 72%,[17,31,32] and therefore should not be solely relied on to differentiate benign from malignant lesions.

VASCULAR PATTERN

The vascular pattern around or within a nodule may correlate with the probability of malignancy. Chammas and colleagues[33] classified thyroid nodules according to the

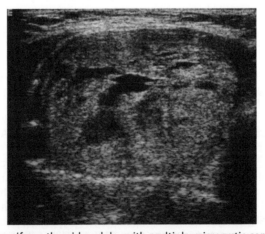

Fig. 3. Benign, spongiform thyroid nodule, with multiple microcystic components.

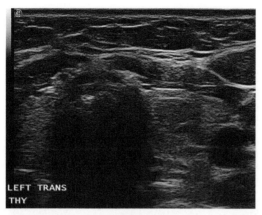

Fig. 4. Slightly hypoechoic benign adenomatous nodule.

pattern of vascularity seen with power Doppler into 5 types: absent blood flow, perinodular flow only, perinodular flow as great or greater than central blood flow, mainly central nodular flow, and central flow only. Nodules with exclusively central blood flow or central blood flow greater than perinodular flow had a higher incidence of malignancy (**Fig. 8**). Follicular carcinomas also tend to show a moderate increase in central vascularity by power Doppler compared with follicular adenomas, which favor peripheral flow (**Fig. 9**).[34] In general, increased vascularity in a thyroid nodule is suggestive of malignancy but should not be considered a pathognomonic feature.

ELASTOGRAPHY

Elastography is the ultrasound measurement of tissue elasticity, a mechanical property reflecting the deformation or distortion of the tissue in response to the application of external compression.[35] In this method, pressure is applied with the ultrasound transducer and used to measure tissue stiffness. The displacement of the strained tissue is estimated by tracking the echo delays in segmented waveforms recorded

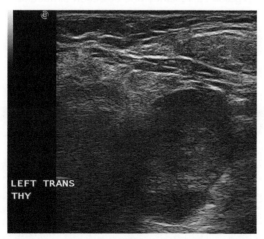

Fig. 5. Moderately hypoechoic and elongated nodule that proved to be a follicular carcinoma.

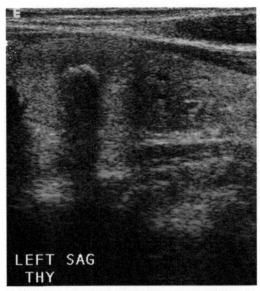

Fig. 6. Peripheral or eggshell calcification in a benign thyroid nodule. Note posterior acoustic shadowing deep to hyperechoic calcification.

before and after quasistatic compression. In vitro studies with various tumors show 10-fold greater stiffness of malignant neoplasms compared with normal tissues.[31] Several studies have investigated the application of ultrasound elastography to thyroid nodules, and found that the sensitivity and specificity of this technique for thyroid cancer diagnosis ranges from 82% to 100% and 81% to 97%, respectively.[31,36,37] Accuracy in one study was approximately 80%.[31] The technique seems to be limited in lesions with coarse calcifications, a significant cystic component, and in differentiating follicular lesions.[31,37] Although the use of this technique remains controversial, lacks standardized measurements for widespread use, and has yet to be prospectively validated, it seems to hold promise in differentiating benign from malignant lesions and may help guide surveillance and selection of nodules for FNA.

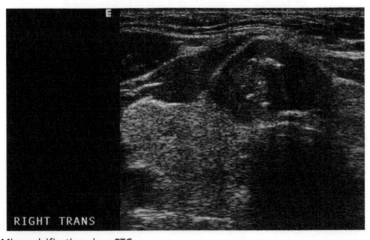

Fig. 7. Microcalcifications in a PTC.

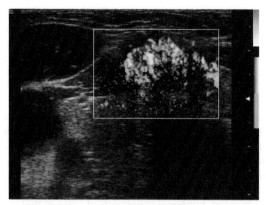

Fig. 8. Increased central blood flow in a papillary carcinoma.

ULTRASOUND CHARACTERISTICS OF MALIGNANT LESIONS

Most thyroid nodules are benign, with approximately 10% of nodules representing malignancy.[38] Risk factors for cancer include female gender, advanced age, exposure to ionizing radiation, and a family history of thyroid cancer. Most thyroid cancers are of follicular cell origin, including papillary, follicular, and Hürthle cell carcinoma, collectively called well-differentiated thyroid cancer. Other malignancies such as MTC, anaplastic carcinoma, lymphoma, and metastatic disease are less common.

As mentioned earlier, ultrasound characteristics of thyroid nodules do not offer sufficient specificity to diagnose malignancy. Regardless, ultrasound represents an invaluable tool in identifying thyroid lesions and aids in determining which lesions should undergo further evaluation through biopsy or other investigations. The next sections discuss specific ultrasound characteristics of thyroid malignancies.

PAPILLARY CARCINOMA

PTC is the most common thyroid malignancy and represents 70% to 80% of all thyroid cancers. Female/male ratio is 2:1 and the peak age at diagnosis is 20 to 30 years.

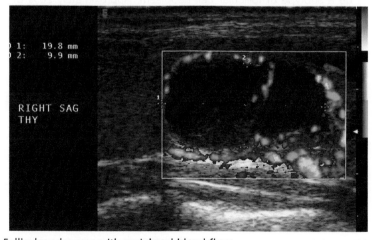

Fig. 9. Follicular adenoma with peripheral blood flow.

Multifocal lesions and regional nodal metastases are common, whereas distant metastases to bone or lung are less common. Local invasion of the larynx, trachea, esophagus, spine, or soft tissues of the neck is seen in only the most aggressive forms of PTC. Prognosis is excellent, with a cure rate up to 90%. Poorer prognosis is associated with large size, advanced patient age, nodal involvement, extrathyroidal spread, male gender, and vascular invasion. Rarely, PTC may degenerate into anaplastic carcinoma.

Ultrasound features typical of PTC include a solid, hypoechoic lesion with microcalcifications (**Fig. 10**). Cystic components may be present within a solid lesion (**Fig. 11**), and although an incomplete halo may be seen, ill-defined margins are more common. Doppler examination may also reveal disorganized hypervascularity. Of these features, microcalcifications may be the most specific for PTC because psammoma bodies are a histopathologic feature considered pathognomonic for PTC; they are composed of tiny laminated, spherical collections of calcium that reflect sound waves and appear as tiny bright foci.

FOLLICULAR CARCINOMA

Follicular carcinoma accounts for approximately 10% of thyroid malignancies. It is more common in older women, has a female/male ratio of 3:1, and has a mean age at diagnosis of 50 years.[39] Unlike PTC, follicular carcinoma is more likely to spread via hematogenous routes, accounting for a higher incidence of distant metastases and poorer prognosis.

Follicular neoplasms, both benign and malignant, typically appear as solid, hypoechoic, and homogenous lesions (**Fig. 12**). Cystic components and calcifications are rare and a halo is often seen. Hypervascularity is common and FNA samples are often bloody. The most important prognostic features are whether vascular, extracapsular, and/or local invasion is present. Because follicular adenoma cannot be distinguished from follicular carcinoma on FNA, the predominance of follicular cells on FNA, especially in sheets or microfollicles, often necessitates an excisional biopsy of the affected lobe.

HÜRTHLE CELL CARCINOMA

The World Health Organization classification of thyroid lesions considers Hürthle cell tumors to be a subtype of follicular cell neoplasm. Approximately 20% of Hürthle

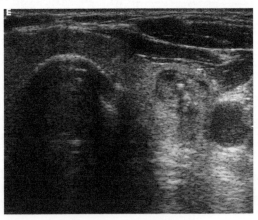

Fig. 10. PTC: solid, hypoechoic lesion with microcalcifications.

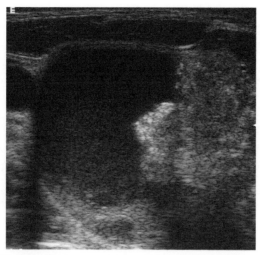

Fig. 11. Cystic papillary carcinoma.

cell lesions are malignant and they account for only 3% of thyroid cancers. These tumors behave more aggressively than either PTC or follicular carcinoma, and often present with bilateral and multifocal lesions, with a higher risk of regional lymph node and distant metastasis.

On ultrasound, Hürthle cell tumors are solid, with both hypoechoic and hyperechoic components with an irregular border (**Fig. 13**). Most do not have calcifications or a halo.

MEDULLARY CARCINOMA

MTCs account for 5% of thyroid cancers. They arise from parafollicular C cells, which are primarily concentrated in the superior poles.[39] Women and men are affected equally, and although most cases are spontaneous, up to 30% are familial and may be associated with multiple endocrine neoplasia (MEN) syndromes type 2A and 2B.

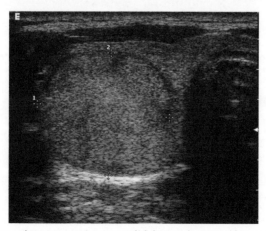

Fig. 12. Follicular neoplasm, appearing as a solid, hypoechoic, and homogenous lesion. This nodule proved to be a follicular adenoma.

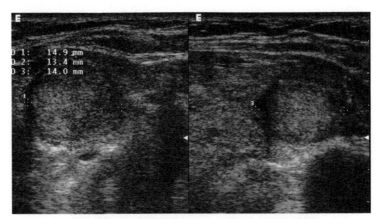

Fig. 13. Hürthle cell adenoma (by histology) that is solid with both hypoechoic and hyperechoic components.

MTC occurring in the setting of an MEN syndrome is usually multifocal and bilateral. Spread to regional lymph nodes in the neck and/or mediastinum and hematogenous spread are common.

MTC appears solid and hypoechoic on ultrasound yet frequently has hyperechoic foci, representing both amyloid deposition and calcification (**Fig. 14**). These foci may also appear within affected lymph nodes. As with papillary carcinoma, Doppler examination may reveal disorganized hypervascularity.[40]

ANAPLASTIC CARCINOMA

Anaplastic carcinoma is the most aggressive type of thyroid cancer. Although it accounts for less than 2% of all thyroid cancers, it comprises up to 40% of deaths from thyroid cancer.[41] It is a disease of elderly people, with few cases occurring in

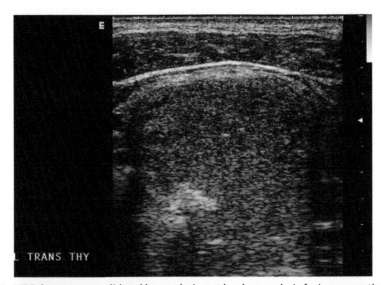

Fig. 14. MTC that appears solid and hypoechoic, yet has hyperechoic foci, representing both amyloid deposition and calcification.

patients younger than 50 years. Most anaplastic carcinomas develop in the setting of a preexisting or coexisting thyroid cancer or goiter and may represent malignant transformation of a previously well-differentiated carcinoma. Patients typically present with a rapidly enlarging neck mass associated with pain, voice changes, dysphagia, or dyspnea. Most patients have lymph node involvement at the time of diagnosis.

Ultrasound shows a diffusely hypoechoic lesion, often infiltrating the entire thyroid lobe, with areas of necrosis or ill-defined calcifications (**Fig. 15**). Involved lymph nodes may also have necrotic changes. Invasion into surrounding vessels or soft tissue is often seen.

LYMPHOMA

Lymphoma involving the thyroid gland is rare, accounting for less than 5% of thyroid malignancies.[41] It may be primary or arise as part of a systemic lymphoma. Women are more often affected and age at diagnosis is usually greater than 50 years. Non-Hodgkin lymphoma is the most common type and is usually associated with a history of Hashimoto thyroiditis. The cytologic diagnosis can be easily mistaken for chronic lymphocytic thyroiditis. The clinical course of thyroid lymphoma may resemble anaplastic carcinoma, with a rapidly enlarging neck mass, regional lymph node enlargement, and symptoms related to compression of the recurrent laryngeal nerve or trachea. However, lymphoma is usually not associated with pain. Local soft-tissue and vascular invasion are both common.

Lymphoma may appear as a focal lesion within a lobe or as a diffuse abnormality involving the entire gland (**Fig. 16**). The involved tissue is usually heterogeneous and hypoechoic and may be mistaken for anaplastic carcinoma. Pseudocysts with posterior enhancement are sometimes seen.

THYROID AS A SITE OF CANCER METASTASES

Metastases to the thyroid gland are uncommon and usually arise from a primary melanoma, breast, lung, or renal cell carcinoma.[39,40] Thyroid metastases usually involve the inferior poles and are homogenous, hypoechoic, and noncalcified.

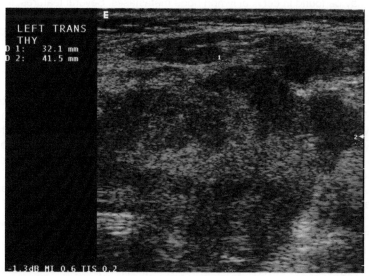

Fig. 15. Anaplastic carcinoma, seen as a diffusely hypoechoic lesion with irregular borders.

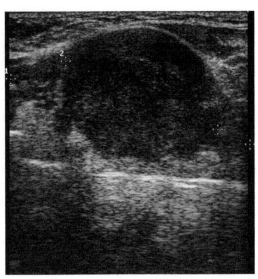

Fig. 16. Lymphoma may appear as a focal heterogeneous and hypoechoic lesion within a background of chronic lymphocytic thyroiditis.

LYMPH NODES

The cervical nodal beds should be evaluated for the presence of abnormally enlarged or otherwise abnormal lymph nodes. Prelaryngeal, pretracheal, and paratracheal (level VI) lymph nodes are a common site of thyroid carcinoma metastasis; however, these nodes are often not amenable to adequate ultrasound evaluation because of thyroid gland obstruction. In contrast, ultrasound is useful and sensitive in the evaluation of lateral cervical lymph nodes and the central (level VI) compartment after thyroidectomy. Ultrasound is also invaluable in the surveillance for recurrent thyroid cancer. The same ultrasound characteristics that are suggestive of malignancy within a thyroid nodule may be found in cervical lymph node metastases. Several features, including cystic appearance, hyperechoic punctuations, loss of hilum, and peripheral vascularization have been associated with malignancy.[42,43] Enlargement, rounded shape, and irregular or indistinct margins can also be seen (**Fig. 17**).[44]

ULTRASOUND SURVEILLANCE OF BENIGN NODULES

Thyroid nodules that appear benign on both cytology and ultrasound should be clinically followed over time. Although malignant transformation of benign thyroid nodules is believed to be rare, there is a 3% to 5% false-negative rate of FNA. Both the ATA and AACE/AME recommend that cytologically benign thyroid nodules be followed every 6 to 18 months with palpation if easily palpable or with ultrasound if not easily palpable.[1,2] The nodules should undergo repeat FNA if there is evidence for nodule growth, defined as a 20% increase in nodule diameter with a minimum increase in 2 or more dimensions of at least 2 mm.[1]

ROLE OF ULTRASOUND IN THYROID GLAND DISEASES
Graves Disease

Palpable thyroid nodules are found 3 times as frequently in patients with Graves disease compared with the general population, and approximately 17% of these

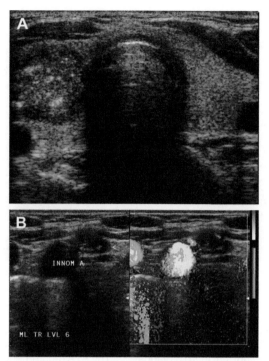

Fig. 17. Similar ultrasound features, including hypoechoic and/or cystic appearance, micro-calcifications, and peripheral vascularization can be seen in this primary PTC in the right thyroid lobe (*A*) and within an adjacent low midline level VI lymph node (*B*). The figure shows a scan in a transverse plane, descending through the thyroid and to the suprasternal level VI, where the metastatic node abuts the innominate artery.

nodules harbor malignancy.[45] A prospective study evaluated patients with Graves disease with physical examination, ultrasound, and scintigraphy; thyroid nodules were identified in 47%, 16%, and 2% of patients, respectively, and 54% of the nodules identified with ultrasound harbored malignancy.[46] The investigators advocate ultrasound examination of all patients with Graves disease.

Ultrasound features of thyroid glands in patients with Graves disease include heterogeneous tissue with diffuse hypoechogenicity and hypervascularity (**Fig. 18**). The velocity of flow in the inferior thyroid artery is typically increased. Color flow mapping may be useful in selecting the optimal dose of antithyroid medication to achieve a euthyroid state,[47] and may also be predictive of the likelihood of relapse after the withdrawal of antithyroid medications.[48,49]

Multinodular Goiter

The risk of malignancy is similar in patients with multiple nodules compared with those with single nodules.[8] The number of nodules present has not been shown to correlate with risk of malignancy.[33] Each nodule should be evaluated independently. In patients with more then one nodule greater than 1 cm, FNA should be guided by ultrasound characteristics suspicious for malignancy rather than size.[1,2] If multiple enlarged nodules are present and none displays suspicious findings on ultrasound, the largest nodules should be sampled and smaller nodules followed with serial ultrasound examinations.[1]

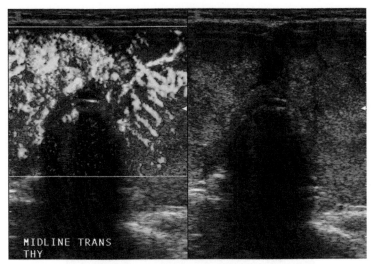

Fig. 18. Thyroid ultrasonography in Graves disease shows thickened heterogeneous parenchyma with diffuse hypoechogenicity and hypervascularity.

Thyroiditis

The rate of malignancy in nodules in patients with Hashimoto thyroiditis is equal to or greater than those in normal thyroid glands.[50,51] The ATA recommends that all patients with an increased level of thyroid-stimulating hormone undergo diagnostic ultrasound.[1] Ultrasound findings include ill-defined hypoechoic areas separated by echogenic septa, with increased or decreased vascularity (**Fig. 19**). Intrathyroid lymphoid tissue accumulates as a result of the autoimmune process in association with thyroid peroxidase antibodies,[52] and patients with Hashimoto thyroiditis have up to a 60-fold increase in the risk of developing lymphoma.[53,54] Chronic lymphocytic thyroiditis is also often associated with central compartment inflammatory lymphadenopathy, which can be difficult to distinguish from small malignant lymphadenopathy.

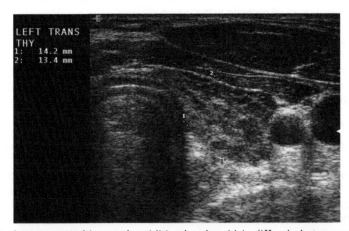

Fig. 19. In late-stage Hashimoto thyroiditis, the thyroid is diffusely heterogeneous and atrophic.

Thyroid Cysts

Cystic nodules represent approximately 20% of all thyroid nodules.[16] Purely cystic lesions are nearly uniformly benign; however, these comprise only 2% of all cystic lesions.[26] Approximately 15% of cystic nodules represent necrotic papillary cancers and 30% represent hemorrhagic adenomas.[9] Most decrease in size over time or completely disappear.[55] Rates of nondiagnostic FNA are high with cystic lesions, and therefore ultrasound-guided FNA is recommended to ensure sampling of the solid component.[1]

SUMMARY: ULTRASOUND AS A TOOL FOR OTOLARYNGOLOGISTS

Thyroid ultrasonography has proved to be an invaluable, first-line tool in the evaluation, management, and treatment of a variety of thyroid disorders. Its indications and uses span both benign and malignant diseases, and continue to expand with improvements in technology. A variety of physicians find benefit by incorporating thyroid ultrasonography into their clinical and operative practice.

REFERENCES

1. Cooper DS, Doherty GM, Haugen BR, et al. Revised American Thyroid Association management guidelines for patients with thyroid nodules and differentiated thyroid cancer. Thyroid 2009;19:1167–214.
2. Gharib H, Papini E, Valcavi R, et al. American Association of Clinical Endocrinologists and Associazione Medici Endocrinologi medical guidelines for clinical practice for the diagnosis and management of thyroid nodules. Endocr Pract 2006;12:63–102.
3. Thijs LG. Diagnostic ultrasound in clinical thyroid investigation. J Clin Endocrinol Metab 1971;32:709–16.
4. Rosen IB, Walfish PG, Miskin M. The application of ultrasound to the study of thyroid enlargement: management of 450 cases. Arch Surg 1975;110:940–4.
5. Spencer R, Brown MC, Annis D. Ultrasonic scanning of the thyroid gland as a guide to the treatment of the clinically solitary nodule. Br J Surg 1977;64:841–6.
6. Lees WR, Vahl SP, Watson LR, et al. The role of ultrasound scanning in the diagnosis of thyroid swellings. Br J Surg 1978;65:681–4.
7. Mortensen JD, Woolner LB, Bennett WA. Gross and microscopic findings in clinically normal thyroid glands. J Clin Endocrinol Metab 1955;15:1270–80.
8. Marqusee E, Benson CB, Frates MC, et al. Usefulness of ultrasonography in the management of nodular thyroid disease. Ann Intern Med 2000;133:696–700.
9. Mazzaferri EL. Management of a solitary thyroid nodule. N Engl J Med 1993;328:553–9.
10. Tunbridge WM, Evered DC, Hall R, et al. The spectrum of thyroid disease in a community: the Whickham survey. Clin Endocrinol (Oxf) 1977;7:481–93.
11. Gharib H, Goellner JR. Fine-needle aspiration biopsy of the thyroid: an appraisal. Ann Intern Med 1993;118:282–9.
12. Cesur M, Corapcioglu D, Bulut S, et al. Comparison of palpation-guided fine-needle aspiration biopsy to ultrasound-guided fine-needle aspiration biopsy in the evaluation of thyroid nodules. Thyroid 2006;16:555–61.
13. Koike E, Yamashita H, Noguchi S, et al. Effect of combining ultrasonography and ultrasound-guided fine-needle aspiration biopsy findings for the diagnosis of thyroid nodules. Eur J Surg 2001;167:656–61.

14. Hatada T, Okada K, Ishii H, et al. Evaluation of ultrasound-guided fine-needle aspiration biopsy for thyroid nodules. Am J Surg 1998;175:133–6.

15. Takashima S, Fukuda H, Kobayashi T. Thyroid nodules: clinical effect of ultrasound-guided fine-needle aspiration biopsy. J Clin Ultrasound 1994;22:535–42.

16. Morris LF, Ragavendra N, Yeh MW. Evidence-based assessment of the role of ultrasonography in the management of benign thyroid nodules. World J Surg 2008;32:1253–63.

17. Cappelli C, Castellano M, Pirola I, et al. The predictive value of ultrasound findings in the management of thyroid nodules. QJM 2007;100:29–35.

18. Kim EK, Park CS, Chung WY, et al. New sonographic criteria for recommending fine-needle aspiration biopsy of nonpalpable solid nodules of the thyroid. AJR Am J Roentgenol 2002;178:687–91.

19. Hagag P, Strauss S, Weiss M. Role of ultrasound-guided fine-needle aspiration biopsy in evaluation of nonpalpable thyroid nodules. Thyroid 1998;8:989–95.

20. Nam-Goong IS, Kim HY, Gong G, et al. Ultrasonography-guided fine-needle aspiration of thyroid incidentaloma: correlation with pathological findings. Clin Endocrinol (Oxf) 2004;60:21–8.

21. Papini E, Guglielmi R, Bianchini A, et al. Risk of malignancy in nonpalpable thyroid nodules: predictive value of ultrasound and color-Doppler features. J Clin Endocrinol Metab 2002;87:1941–6.

22. Ultrasonography of the Thyroid. Thyroid disease manager, Ch. 6C. Available at: http://www.thyroidmanager.org. Accessed November 20, 2009.

23. Baskin HJ. Thyroid ultrasound and ultrasound-guided FNA biopsy. Norwell (MA): Kluwer Academic Publishers; 2000.

24. Koike E, Noguchi S, Yamashita H, et al. Ultrasonographic characteristics of thyroid nodules: prediction of malignancy. Arch Surg 2001;136:334–7.

25. Leenhardt L, Menegaux F, Franc B, et al. Selection of patients with solitary thyroid nodules for operation. Eur J Surg 2002;168:236–41.

26. Frates MC, Benson CB, Doubilet PM, et al. Prevalence and distribution of carcinoma in patients with solitary and multiple thyroid nodules on sonography. J Clin Endocrinol Metab 2006;91:3411–7.

27. Moon WJ, Jung SL, Lee JH, et al. Benign and malignant thyroid nodules: US differentiation–multicenter retrospective study. Radiology 2008;247:762–70.

28. Bonavita JA, Mayo J, Babb J, et al. Pattern recognition of benign nodules at ultrasound of the thyroid: which nodules can be left alone? AJR Am J Roentgenol 2009;193:207–13.

29. Kang HW, No JH, Chung JH, et al. Prevalence, clinical and ultrasonographic characteristics of thyroid incidentalomas. Thyroid 2004;14:29–33.

30. Seiberling KA, Dutra JC, Grant T, et al. Role of intrathyroidal calcifications detected on ultrasound as a marker of malignancy. Laryngoscope 2004;114:1753–7.

31. Asteria C, Giovanardi A, Pizzocaro A, et al. US-elastography in the differential diagnosis of benign and malignant thyroid nodules. Thyroid 2008;18:523–31.

32. Iannuccilli JD, Cronan JJ, Monchik JM. Risk for malignancy of thyroid nodules as assessed by sonographic criteria: the need for biopsy. J Ultrasound Med 2004; 23:1455–64.

33. Chammas MC, Gerhard R, de Oliveira IR, et al. Thyroid nodules: evaluation with power Doppler and duplex Doppler ultrasound. Otolaryngol Head Neck Surg 2005;132:874–82.

34. Miyakawa M, Onoda N, Etoh M, et al. Diagnosis of thyroid follicular carcinoma by the vascular pattern and velocimetric parameters using high resolution pulsed and power Doppler ultrasonography. Endocr J 2005;52:207–12.

35. Chaturvedi P, Insana MF, Hall TJ. Ultrasonic and elasticity imaging to model disease-induced changes in soft-tissue structure. Med Image Anal 1998;2: 325–38.
36. Rago T, Santini F, Scutari M, et al. Elastography: new developments in ultrasound for predicting malignancy in thyroid nodules. J Clin Endocrinol Metab 2007;92: 2917–22.
37. Lyshchik A, Higashi T, Asato R, et al. Thyroid gland tumor diagnosis at US elastography. Radiology 2005;237:202–11.
38. Mandel SJ. A 64-year-old woman with a thyroid nodule. JAMA 2004;292:2632–42.
39. Cummings CW, Haughey B, Thomas JR, et al. Cummings otolaryngology – head and neck surgery. 4th edition. St Louis (MO): Mosby; 2005.
40. Ahuja A. Practical head and neck ultrasound. London: Greenwich Medical Media; 2000.
41. Green LD, Mack L, Pasieka JL. Anaplastic thyroid cancer and primary thyroid lymphoma: a review of these rare thyroid malignancies. J Surg Oncol 2006;94: 725–36.
42. Leboulleux S, Girard E, Rose M, et al. Ultrasound criteria of malignancy for cervical lymph nodes in patients followed up for differentiated thyroid cancer. J Clin Endocrinol Metab 2007;92:3590–4.
43. Rosario PW, de Faria S, Bicalho L, et al. Ultrasonographic differentiation between metastatic and benign lymph nodes in patients with papillary thyroid carcinoma. J Ultrasound Med 2005;24:1385–9.
44. Orloff LA. Head and neck ultrasonography. San Diego (CA): Plural Publishing; 2008.
45. Belfiore A, Russo D, Vigneri R, et al. Graves' disease, thyroid nodules and thyroid cancer. Clin Endocrinol (Oxf) 2001;55:711–8.
46. Cappelli C, Pirola I, De Martino E, et al. The role of imaging in Graves' disease: a cost-effectiveness analysis. Eur J Radiol 2008;65:99–103.
47. Saleh A, Furst G, Feldkamp J, et al. Estimation of antithyroid drug dose in Graves' disease: value of quantification of thyroid blood flow with color duplex sonography. Ultrasound Med Biol 2001;27:1137–41.
48. Saleh A, Cohnen M, Furst G, et al. Prediction of relapse after antithyroid drug therapy of Graves' disease: value of color Doppler sonography. Exp Clin Endocrinol Diabetes 2004;112:510–3.
49. Varsamidis K, Varsamidou E, Mavropoulos G. Doppler ultrasonography in predicting relapse of hyperthyroidism in Graves' disease. Acta Radiol 2000;41:45–8.
50. Singh B, Shaha AR, Trivedi H, et al. Coexistent Hashimoto's thyroiditis with papillary thyroid carcinoma: impact on presentation, management, and outcome. Surgery 1999;126:1070–6 [discussion: 1076–7].
51. Repplinger D, Bargren A, Zhang YW, et al. Is Hashimoto's thyroiditis a risk factor for papillary thyroid cancer? J Surg Res 2008;150:49–52.
52. Thieblemont C, Mayer A, Dumontet C, et al. Primary thyroid lymphoma is a heterogeneous disease. J Clin Endocrinol Metab 2002;87:105–11.
53. Kato I, Tajima K, Suchi T, et al. Chronic thyroiditis as a risk factor of B-cell lymphoma in the thyroid gland. Jpn J Cancer Res 1985;76:1085–90.
54. Holm LE, Blomgren H, Lowhagen T. Cancer risks in patients with chronic lymphocytic thyroiditis. N Engl J Med 1985;312:601–4.
55. Kuma K, Matsuzuka F, Yokozawa T, et al. Fate of untreated benign thyroid nodules: results of long-term follow-up. World J Surg 1994;18:495–8 [discussion: 499].

Techniques for Parathyroid Localization with Ultrasound

Lisa Lee, MD, David L. Steward, MD*

KEYWORDS

- Parathyroid adenoma • Parathyroid localization
- Ultrasonography

PARATHYROID WORKUP

Four-gland parathyroid exploration has been the gold standard for parathyroid surgery until recently. Emphasis is now placed on minimally invasive and focused parathyroidectomy. Given this objective, there is a need for sensitive and accurate localization of parathyroid pathology. Effective imaging techniques are instrumental in achieving these ends, particularly in the midst of heightened awareness of cost containment.

A thorough medical workup identifies the cause underlying hypercalcemia in the vast majority of patients. Hyperparathyroidism accounts for most cases of hypercalcemia and is categorized as primary, secondary, or tertiary. Primary hyperparathyroidism is the most common cause of hypercalcemia, affecting an estimated 0.2% to 0.5% of the US population. There are approximately 100,000 new cases each year.[1] One in 500 women and one in 2000 men usually in their fifties to seventies are affected.[2] Clinical manifestations of hypercalcemia include fatigue, hypertension, bone pain, muscle weakness, renal stones, peptic ulcers, and psychiatric illness.[2,3] Laboratory abnormalities include hypercalcemia, hypophosphatemia, elevated parathyroid hormone levels, and increased urine calcium excretion. Secondary hyperparathyroidism is usually found in patients with renal insufficiency marked by hypocalcemia and hyperphosphatemia or in the setting of vitamin D deficiency. Tertiary hyperparathyroidism occurs with the development of autonomously hyperfunctioning parathyroid glands of secondary hyperparathyroidism with resultant hypercalcemia.[4–7]

Primary hyperparathyroidism may be sporadic or hereditary, with sporadic being much more common. Spontaneous primary hyperparathyroidism is most often due

Department of Otolaryngology-Head and Neck Surgery, University of Cincinnati Medical Center, Medical Sciences Building, Room 6507, 231 Albert Sabin Way, Cincinnati, OH 45267-0582, USA
* Corresponding author.
E-mail address: david.steward@uc.edu

Otolaryngol Clin N Am 43 (2010) 1229–1239
doi:10.1016/j.otc.2010.08.002
0030-6665/10/$ – see front matter © 2010 Elsevier Inc. All rights reserved.

to solitary parathyroid adenomas (85 to 90%), 4-gland hyperplasia (10 to 15%) or multiple adenomas, or asymmetric hyperplasia (2 to 3%) but rarely due to parathyroid carcinoma (less than 1%).[3,8–10] Hereditary primary hyperparathyroidism may be isolated, associated with jaw tumor syndrome or other endocrine neoplasia. In hereditary primary hyperparathyroidism, multigland disease (multiple endocrine neoplasia 1 or 2a) is the rule rather than the exception.[11]

Identification and localization of parathyroid adenomas is crucial for selective parathyroid surgery. Previously, the predominant localization technique involved sestamibi scanning. Its limitations have prompted investigations for more effective tools, including ultrasound technology. Unlike sestamibi scanning, ultrasonography offers more precise anatomic localization with concomitant facilitation of surgical planning.

ULTRASONOGRAPHY IN THE PARATHYROID WORKUP

In the setting of primary hyperparathyroidism, one study found that ultrasonography had a sensitivity, specificity, and positive predictive value of 60%, 91%, and 92%, respectively, in detecting adenomas.[12] In the authors' experience of surgically proven adenomas, ultrasound sensitivity was 90%, better than sestamibi (70%).[13] Ultrasonography is a much less sensitive tool for identifying hyperplasia.[14] In the setting of secondary hyperparathyroidism, ultrasound had a sensitivity of 60% and accuracy of 64% in localizing enlarged parathyroid glands, missing as many as 30% of patients with multigland disease.[12,15] Furthermore, patients with negative localization by scintigraphy and ultrasound were more likely to have 4-gland hyperplasia.

The accuracy of ultrasonography is also affected by thyroid disease, because its sensitivity dropped from 100% to 84% to 93% and positive predictive value decreased from 100% to 84%.[16–18] Nodular thyroid disease may also contribute to false-positive or negative results. Infrathyroidal lymph nodes associated with thyroiditis may result in a false-positive interpretation as inferior adenomas. Decreased sensitivity is often a consequence of poor echogenic differentiation of parathyroid tissue.

ANATOMY & EMBRYOLOGY

Most individuals have 4 parathyroid glands (80%), 2 superior and 2 inferior. Supernumerary fifth or sixth glands may be found in 13% to 25% of the population, whereas 3% to 5% of the population has fewer than 4 parathyroid glands.[4,19–22] Approximately 1% to 3% of parathyroid glands are ectopic.[19,22]

The superior parathyroid glands arise from the fourth branchial pouch. They descend the neck in an inferoposterior direction to reside posterior to the recurrent laryngeal nerve, a sixth arch derivative. Most superior parathyroid glands are located posterior to the middle or upper portion of the thyroid gland in the vicinity of the cricothyroid junction. Less commonly, they may be located inferior to the midportion of the thyroid lobe (4%) or above the superior pole of the thyroid gland (3%). Occasionally, superior parathyroid glands may migrate toward the tracheoesophageal groove or the posterior mediastinum. Such ectopic adenomas account for less than 3% and may be found in the retropharyngeal, retroesophageal, posterior paratracheal, or intrathyroidal spaces.[19,22–26]

The inferior parathyroid glands arise from the third branchial pouch. They descend the neck in an inferoanterior direction, often in close association with the thymus, and eventually reside anterior to the recurrent laryngeal nerve. Because the inferior parathyroid glands travel a greater distance, there is more variability in their final position. They may be found anywhere from the hyoid bone to the pericardium. More often, they are located inferior or just posterior to the lower pole of the thyroid, near the inferior thyroid artery (45%–60%).[19,22,23,25,26]

Ectopic inferior parathyroid glands may be found in the cervical thymus (26%), anterosuperior mediastinum within the thymus (2%), or inferior to the thymus deep in the mediastinum (0.2%). Alternatively, the inferior parathyroid glands may fail to adequately descend and consequently remain cephalad to the superior glands. Ectopic glands within the carotid sheath may be surrounded by thymic fat. They may also be recognized within the inferior pole of the thyroid gland.[21,27–29]

SONOGRAPHIC APPEARANCE OF THE PARATHYROID GLANDS

Normal parathyroid glands are rarely visualized, because of their small size and insufficient acoustic difference from surrounding tissue. The average size of a normal parathyroid gland is $5 \times 3 \times 1$ mm, with a range of 2 to 12 mm. Each gland usually weighs an average of 40 mg with a range of 10 to 78 mg.[14,22,23,25] In contrast, parathyroid adenomas, hyperplasia, and carcinomas exhibit a relatively hypoechogenic pattern, because of their compact cellularity relative to thyroid tissue.[18] Hyperplastic glands in primary hyperparathyroidism are often 2 to 4 times larger than normal. However, hyperplastic parathyroids are difficult to detect unless they exhibit a significant increase in total gland volume. Microcalcifications may be present in hyperplasia, particularly in patients with secondary hyperparathyroidism.[14] Enlarged parathyroids with indistinct borders suggest a carcinoma.[30–32]

Parathyroid adenomas are usually well-circumscribed ovoid, bilobed, polygonal, triangular, or longitudinal in shape. They tend to be solid and homogenously hypoechoic relative to echogenic thyroid tissue.[9,10,19,20,33] Overall, the ability to detect a parathyroid adenoma is a function of its size. The smaller the adenoma, the more difficult the task of localizing it radiographically. The lower limit of detection was reported to be 4 to 8 mm, with a 90% accurate rate of diagnosis in glands weighing more than 500 mg, although the authors often detect small adenomas down to 100 to 200 mg.[13,34,35] The average mass of parathyroid adenomas is 10 times greater than normal parathyroid glands.[36–38] Rarely, cystic changes or calcifications may be seen in adenomas undergoing complete or partial cystic degeneration.[33,39–42] Seldom encountered, lipoadenomas appear hyperechoic because of increased fat content within the parathyroid adenoma.[43]

SONOGRAPHIC TECHNIQUE

To begin the ultrasonographic examination, the patient is placed in a comfortable, semireclined position facing midline, with the neck mildly extended. Neck extension allows slight elevation of mediastinal structures out of the thoracic inlet and may be exaggerated for mediastinal imaging. In most patients, a high frequency linear transducer may be used (8 to 15 MHz). Examination of larger patients may require a lower frequency to allow adequate sonographic penetration.

The proper frequency setting should allow optimal spatial resolution while also enabling adequate tissue penetration to visualize deep structures, such as the prevertebral musculature. Increasing the far-field or overall gain may also improve detection of deep parathyroid glands by facilitating the sonographic difference between prevertebral musculature and parathyroid tissue.[7,21,44–48]

Ultrasonographic examination ideally follows a routine pathway, focusing on one side of the neck at a time in a slow and deliberate fashion. Initial evaluation involves the central neck compartment, focusing between the carotid arteries laterally and trachea medially. Starting in the transverse plane at the level of the innominate vessels inferiorly, scanning can progress superiorly to the superior pole of the thyroid or hyoid. The transducer is then moved in a lateral to medial direction for longitudinal scanning. Although longitudinal scanning is initially more challenging, it is necessary to corroborate abnormalities detected in the transverse plane and to detect adenomas missed with transverse scanning.

Skin and subcutaneous fat is first encountered by sound waves. Beneath these layers, the strap muscles (sternohyoid, omohyoid, and sternothyroid) centrally and sternocleidomastoid muscle laterally are visualized.

Muscle tissue may be distinguished by its fibrillar hypoechoic appearance compared with the echogenic texture of thyroid tissue. The thyroid gland may be assessed for nodules and microcalcifications among other features.

The esophagus may be found to the left side of the trachea. It has a hypoechoic peripheral muscular layer and an echogenic central mucosa. It may be better identified on dynamic imaging while observing the patient swallow. The prevertebral musculature is seen posterior to the thyroid gland.

Laterally in the neck, the contents of the carotid sheath may be seen adjacent to the thyroid gland. A distinction between the artery and vein can be made based on the compressibility of venous structures and more anterior and lateral position of the internal jugular vein.

The central neck is first evaluated for orthotopic parathyroid glands, with particular attention to the common locations aforementioned. The superior gland is commonly found posterior to the middle third of the thyroid gland and sometimes in the trachea-esophageal groove, (**Fig. 1**) demonstrate the location of an orthotopic superior parathyroid gland. The inferior gland usually lies near the inferior pole of the thyroid gland, (**Fig. 2**) demonstrate the location of an orthotopic inferior parathyroid gland.

If an adenoma is not identified after scanning the central neck in the transverse and longitudinal planes, then a systematic search for common ectopic locations is conducted. Common ectopic locations for superior parathyroid glands are retroesophageal, deep inferior mediastinum, and, occasionally, posterior intrathyroidal.

Common ectopic locations for inferior parathyroid glands are inferior intrathyroidal, intrathymic, carotid sheath, or anterior mediastinum. Intrathyroidal parathyroid glands may be differentiated from thyroid nodules or thyroid parenchyma by their relatively hypoechoic signal; however, differentiation may require ultrasound-guided fine-needle aspiration (FNA) for cytology, staining, and parathyroid hormone assay of needle-wash contents.

An enlarged gland in the paraesophageal region may pop into view by having patients turn their head away from the side being examined and then swallowing. A hypoechoic mass will be visible along a backdrop of a longitudinally directed muscle. Also, aiming the transducer medially aids in the evaluation of the retrotracheal or paratracheal region; however, retrotracheal ectopic glands may be difficult to detect because of the poor acoustic window caused by the tracheal air column.

A more lateral position of the transducer may decrease the shadow artifact related to the carotid artery and trachea, when examining the central compartment posterior to the carotid artery and trachea.

Tilting the transducer probe is a good adjunct technique to moving the transducer during scanning. To assist in visualization of deeply inferior parathyroid glands, the patient swallows while the ultrasound probe is aimed inferiorly underneath the clavicles. Despite swallowing maneuvers, visualization of mediastinal glands is often difficult because of poor penetration by sound waves.[21,44–47,49,50]

The distinction between superior and inferior parathyroid glands can be occasionally difficult. The key distinguishing feature is based on embryologic origin. Superior

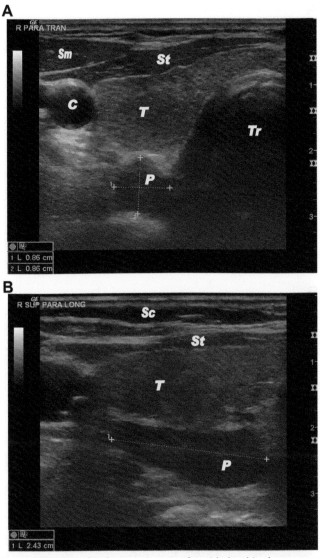

Fig. 1. (*A*) Ultrasound image of right superior parathyroid gland in the transverse plane. (*B*) Ultrasound image of right superior parathyroid gland in the longitudinal plane. C, Carotid artery; P, Parathyroid gland; P, Parathyroid gland; Sm, Sternocleidomastoid muscle; St, Strap muscle; T, Thyroid gland; Tr, Trachea; Sc, Subcutaneous tissue; St, Strap muscle; T, Thyroid gland.

parathyroid glands lie in a deeper plane than inferior parathyroid glands. Superior parathyroid glands lie posterior to the plane of the recurrent laryngeal nerve. The posterior surface of the common carotid artery or the inferior thyroid artery may be used as surrogate markers for the recurrent laryngeal nerve. Hence, an adenoma located entirely deep to these landmarks is most likely a superior parathyroid gland, even if located more inferiorly from its usual orthotopic location.

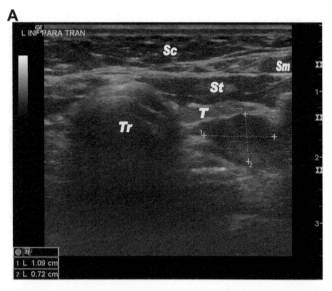

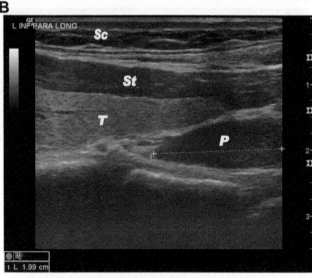

Fig. 2. (*A*) Ultrasound image of left inferior parathyroid gland in the transverse plane. Note the relative homogenous hypoechoic appearance of parathyroid tissue relative to echogenic appearance of thyroid tissue. (*B*) Ultrasound image of left inferior parathyroid gland in the longitudinal plane. Note the elongated, relative homogenous hypoechoic appearance of parathyroid tissue relative to echogenic appearance of thyroid tissue. P, Parathyroid gland; Sc, subcutaneous tissue; Sm, sternocleidomastoid muscle; St, strap muscle; Tr, trachea; T, thyroid gland.

DIFFERENTIATING PARATHYROID GLANDS

Any potential candidate for a parathyroid adenoma must be confirmed in 2 views, in longitudinal and transverse planes, to avoid the pitfalls of false-positive examinations. Normal anatomic structures may be mistaken for parathyroid tissue. Thyroid nodules, enlarged lymph nodes, esophagus, longus colli, and small vessels may be inadvertently mistaken for parathyroid lesions.[51]

Thyroid gland abnormalities may obscure adequate visualization of parathyroid pathology. The sensitivity of high-frequency ultrasound decreases in patients with thyroid nodules compared with patients without thyroid pathology, reducing from 85% to 100% sensitivity to 47% to 84%.[12,17,52,53] In the setting of multinodular goiter, parathyroid adenomas may be overlooked because of poor sonographic penetration, dispersion of the sound waves, or difficulty distinguishing the parathyroid capsule because of the goitrous contour. Alternatively, thyroid nodules may be mistaken for parathyroid adenomas, particularly if they are located posteriorly on the thyroid capsule, (**Fig. 3**) demonstrates a thyroid nodule which may be mistaken for a parathyroid gland.[54,55] Swallowing maneuvers sometimes help differentiate extrathyroidal adenomas from the thyroid gland.

Lymph nodes may be mistaken for adenomas because of their size, location, and appearance, especially in the setting of thyroiditis. Distinguishing between lymph node and parathyroid gland may be more difficult in an older patient, because parathyroid glands tend to accumulate more fat and hence take on a more echogenic appearance.

Prevertebral muscles, veins, or esophagus may be mistaken for adenomas if scanned only in a transverse fashion.[9,56] On transverse view, the esophagus may be mistaken for a posterior parathyroid on the left side. However, a longitudinal view would show its tubular appearance. Peristalsis may also be demonstrated on longitudinal view. The longus colli muscle can be more definitively identified on longitudinal scanning.

In addition to transverse and longitudinal gray-scale sonographic views, graded compression and color Doppler features may be occasionally useful supplementary tools. Graded compression of superficial tissue, such as subcutaneous fat and neck musculature, helps image patients with thick necks. It also may discern small adenomas (<1 cm) from surrounding tissue, particularly in the tracheoesophageal groove or along the longus colli.[44] Color Doppler provides information that aids in differentiating parathyroid glands from lymph nodes and thyroid nodules.[27,57] Its use was

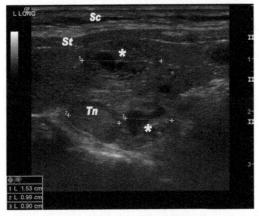

Fig. 3. Ultrasound image of left thyroid lobe with multiple thyroid nodules in the longitudinal plane. The posterior Tn resembles a parathyroid gland. Note the heterogenous appearance of thyroid nodules (*). Sc, subcutaneous tissue; St, strap muscle; Tn, thyroid nodule; *, thyroid nodule.

found to improve sensitivity of parathyroid adenoma detection from 73% to 83%.[46] Color Doppler ultrasound may help identify adenomas by determining the presence of an asymmetric, arclike peripheral hypervascularity.[10,18,45–47,49] In contrast, lymph nodes have a distinct hyperechogenic fatty hilum with a central hilar branching vascular flow pattern. This represents a key distinction, because parathyroid adenomas have a feeding artery with a polar insertion on the long axis.[18,45–47,58]

ULTRASONOGRAPHY SHORTCOMINGS

Ultrasonography as a diagnostic tool is highly dependent on operator skill and patient factors. It also requires a high degree of familiarity with cervical anatomy and knowledge of relative echogenicity of various tissues. Successful ultrasonography requires familiarity with the ultrasound machine, including the use of varying frequencies, gain manipulation, graded compression, and color Doppler. In experienced hands, 70% to 90% of enlarged parathyroid glands can be located.[2,13,56,59] Patient body mass index and neck thickness affect penetration of sound waves.[35] Concomitant thyroid disease makes evaluation of parathyroids more challenging. Limited sound-wave resolution leads to inability to reliably detect small parathyroid glands and to mistake lymph nodes for parathyroid glands.

ULTRASOUND APPLIED TO PARATHYROID PATHOLOGY

Ultrasonography provides cost-effective, convenient, and accurate localization of enlarged parathyroid glands in the vast majority of patients with hyperparathyroidism in conjunction with functional sestamibi scanning. Unlike sestamibi scanning, computed tomography, or other imaging technologies, ultrasonography provides dynamic imaging in the hands of the surgeon who has intimate knowledge of cervical anatomy. The knowledge of exact gland location allows the surgeon to focus tissue exploration and consequently decrease chances of injury to significant structures. Particularly with the advent of intraoperative parathyroid hormone levels, focused minimally invasive parathyroidectomy leads to decreased operative time and reduced morbidity as compared with traditional 4-gland exploration.[56,60,61] Novel applications of parathyroid ultrasonography have also evolved to include ultrasound-guided FNA of suspected intrathyroidal parathyroid glands.[16,39,54,62] Also, percutaneous ethanol ablation of hyperplastic parathyroid glands has been applied to chronic dialysis patients.[63] Ultrasound technology applied to parathyroid pathology facilitates directed surgical therapy and minimally invasive applications and consequently holds great promise as a tool that enables cost-effective and advanced patient care.

REFERENCES

1. Zanocco K, Angelos P, Sturgeon C. Cost-effectiveness analysis of parathyroidectomy for asymptomatic primary hyperparathyroidism. Surgery 2006;140(6): 874–81.
2. Uden P, Chan A, Duy QY, et al. Primary hyperparathyroidism in younger and older patients: symptoms and outcome of surgery. World J Surg 1992;16:791–7.
3. Ruda JM, Hollenbeak CS, Stack BC Jr. A systematic review of the diagnosis and treatment of primary hyperparathyroidism from 1995 to 2003. Otolaryngol Head Neck Surg 2005;132:359–72.
4. Kaplan EL, Yashiro T, Gslti G. Primary hyperparathyroidism in the 1990's. Ann Surg 1992;215:300–17.

5. Pham TH, Sterioff S, Mullan BP, et al. Sensitivity and utility of parathyroid scintig-raphy in patients with primary versus secondary and tertiary hyperparathy-roidism. World J Surg 2006;30(3):327–32.

6. Ahmad R, Hammond JM. Primary, secondary, and tertiary hyperparathyroidism. Otolaryngol Clin North Am 2004;37(4):701–13.

7. Kamaya A, Quon A, Jeffrey RB. Sonography of the abnormal parathyroid gland. Ultrasound Q 2006;22(4):253–62.

8. Kebebew E. Predictors of single-gland vs multigland parathyroid disease in primary hyperparathyroidism: a simple and accurate scoring model. Arch Surg 2006;141(8):777–82.

9. Hopkins CR, Reading CC. Thyroid and parathyroid imaging. Semin Ultrasound CT MR 1995;16(4):279–95.

10. Solbiati L, Osti V, Cova L, et al. Ultrasound of thyroid, parathyroid glands and neck lymph nodes. Eur Radiol 2001;11(12):2411–24.

11. Muhr C, Ljunghall S, Akerstrom G, et al. Screening for multiple endocrine neoplasia syndrome (type 1) in patients with primary hyperparathyroidism. Clin Endocrinol 1984;20:153–62.

12. Sukan A, Reyhan M, Aydin M, et al. Preoperative evaluation of hyperparathy-roidism: the role of dual-phase parathyroid scintigraphy and ultrasound imaging. Ann Nucl Med 2008;22(2):123–31.

13. Steward DL, Danielson GP, Afman CE, et al. Parathyroid adenoma localization: surgeon-performed ultrasound versus sestamibi. Laryngoscope 2006;116(8): 1380–4.

14. Mollerup CL, Bollerslev J, Blichert-Toft M. Primary hyperparathyroidism: inci-dence and clinical and biochemical characteristics—a demographic study. Eur J Surg 1994;160:485–9.

15. Bhansali A, Masoodi SR, Bhadada S, et al. Ultrasonography in detection of single and multiple abnormal parathyroid glands in primary hyperparathyroidism: comparison with radionuclide scintigraphy and surgery. Clin Endocrinol (Oxf) 2006;65(3):340–5.

16. Erbil Y, Salmaslioğlu A, Kabul E, et al. Use of preoperative parathyroid fine-needle aspiration and parathormone assay in the primary hyperparathyroidism with concomitant thyroid nodules. Am J Surg 2007;193(6):665–71.

17. Erbil Y, Barbaros U, Yanik BT, et al. Impact of gland morphology and concomitant thyroid nodules on preoperative localization of parathyroid adenomas. Laryngo-scope 2006;116(4):580–5.

18. Gilat H, Cohen M, Feinmesser R, et al. Minimally invasive procedure for resection of a parathyroid adenoma: the role of preoperative high-resolution ultrasonog-raphy. J Clin Ultrasound 2005;33(6):283–7.

19. WangCA. The anatomic basis of parathyroid surgery. Ann Surg 1976;183: 271–5.

20. Reading CC, Charboneau JW, James EM, et al. High-resolution parathyroid sonography. AJR Am J Roentgenol 1982;139:539.

21. Gooding GA. Sonography of the thyroid and parathyroid. Radiol Clin North Am 1993;31:967.

22. Akerstrom G, Malmaeus J, Bergstrom R. Surgical anatomy of human parathyroid glands. Surgery 1984;95:14.

23. Mansberger AR, Wei JP. Surgical embryology and anatomy of the thyroid and parathyroid glands. Surg Clin North Am 1993;73:727.

24. Weller GLJ. Development of the thyroid, parathyroid and thymus glands in man. Contrib Embryol 1933;24:93.

25. Grimelius L, Bondeson L. Histopathological diagnosis of parathyroid diseases. Pathol Res Pract 1995;191:353–65.
26. Kang YS, Rosen K, Clark OH, et al. Localization of abnormal parathyroid glands of the mediastinum with MR imaging. Radiology 1993;189(1):137–41.
27. Thompson NW, Eckhauser FE, Harness JK. The anatomy of primary hyperparathyroidism. Surgery 1982;92:814.
28. Edis AJ, Purnell DC, van Heerden JA. The undescended "parathymus". An occasional cause of failed neck exploration for hyperparathyroidism. Ann Surg 1979; 190:64.
29. Edis AJ. Surgical anatomy and technique of neck exploration for primary hyperparathyroidism. Surg Clin North Am 1977;57:495.
30. Edmonson GR, Charboneau JW, James EM, et al. Parathyroid carcinoma: High-frequency sonographic features. Radiology 1986;161:65–7.
31. Smith JF, Coombs RRH. Histological diagnosis of carcinoma of the parathyroid gland. J Clin Pathol 1984;37:1370–8.
32. Kinoshita Y, Fukase M, Uchihashi M, et al. Significance of preoperative use of ultrasonography in parathyroid neoplasms: comparison of sonographic textures with histologic findings. J Clin Ultrasound 1985;13(7):457–60.
33. Randel SB, Gooding GA, Clark OH, et al. Parathyroid variants: US evaluation. Radiology 1987;165(1):191–4.
34. Kawata R, Kotetsu L, Takamaki A, et al. Ultrasonography for preoperative localization of enlarged parathyroid glands in secondary hyperparathyroidism. Auris Nasus Larynx 2009;36(4):461–5.
35. Berber E, Parikh RT, Ballem N, et al. Factors contributing to negative parathyroid localization: an analysis of 1000 patients. Surgery 2008;144(1):74–9.
36. Soon PS, Delbridge LW, Sywak MS, et al. Surgeon performed ultrasound facilitates minimally invasive parathyroidectomy by the focused lateral mini-incision approach. World J Surg 2008;32:766–71.
37. Yao K, Singer FR, Roth SI, et al. Weight of normal parathyroid glands in patients with parathyroid adenomas. J Clin Endocrinol Metab 2004;89:3208–13.
38. Tresoldi S, Pompili G, Maiolino R, et al. Primary hyperparathyroidism: can ultrasonography be the only preoperative diagnostic procedure? Radiol Med 2009;114: 1159–72.
39. Silverman JF, Yhazanie PG, Norris HT, et al. Parathyroid hormone (PTH) assay of parathyroid cysts examined by fine-needle aspiration biopsy. Am J Clin Pathol 1986;86:776–80.
40. Graif M, Itzchak Y, Strauss S, et al. Parathyroid sonography: diagnostic accuracy related to shape, location, and texture of the gland. Br J Radiol 1987;60(713):439–43.
41. Lack EF, Clark MA, Buck DR, et al. Cysts of the parathyroid gland: report of two cases and review of the literature. Am Surg 1978;44:376.
42. Krudy AG, Doppman JL, Shawker TH, et al. Hyperfunctioning cystic parathyroid glands: computed tomography and sonographic findings. AJR Am J Roentgenol 1984;142:175.
43. Obara T, Fujimoto Y, Ito Y. Functioning parathyroid lipoadenoma-report of four cases: clinicopathological and ultrasonographic features. Endocrinol Jpn 1989; 36:135.
44. American Institute of Ultrasound in Medicine. AIUM practice guideline for the performance of a thyroid and parathyroid ultrasound examination. J Ultrasound Med 2003;22:1126–30.
45. Reeder SB, Desser TS, Weigel RJ, et al. Sonography in hyperparathyroidism: review with emphasis on scanning technique. J Ultrasound Med 2002;21:539.

46. Lane MJ, Desser TS, Weigel RJ, et al. Use of color and power Doppler sonography to identify feeding arteries associated with parathyroid adenomas. AJR Am J Roentgenol 1998;171:819.
47. Wolf RJ, Cronan JJ, Monchik JM. Color Doppler sonography: an adjunctive technique in assessment of parathyroid adenomas. J Ultrasound Med 1994;13:303.
48. Yeh MW, Barraclough BM, Sidhu SB, et al. Two hundred consecutive parathyroid ultrasound studies by a single clinician: the impact of experience. Endocr Pract 2006;12(3):257–63.
49. Doppman JL, Skarulis MC, Chen CC, et al. Parathyroid adenomas in the aortopulmonary window. Radiology 1996;201(2):456–62.
50. Barraclough BM, Barraclough BH. Ultrasound of the thyroid and parathyroid glands. World J Surg 2000;24(2):158–65.
51. Huppert BJ, Reading CC. Parathyroid sonography: imaging and intervention. J Clin Ultrasound 2007;35(3):144–55.
52. Barbaros U, Erbil Y, Salmashoğlu A, et al. The characteristics of concomitant thyroid nodules cause false-positive ultrasonography results in primary hyperparathyroidism. Am J Otolaryngol 2009;30(4):239–43.
53. Ghaheri BA, Koslin DB, Wood AH, et al. Preoperative ultrasound is worthwhile for reoperative parathyroid surgery. Laryngoscope 2004;114:2168–71.
54. Barczynski M, Golkowski F, Konturek A, et al. Technetium-99m-sestamibi subtraction scintigraphy vs. ultrasonography combined with a rapid parathyroid hormone assay in parathyroid aspirates in preoperative localization of parathyroid adenomas and in directing surgical approach. Clin Endocrinol (Oxf) 2006; 65(1):106–13.
55. Heizmann O, Viehl CT, Schmid R, et al. Impact of concomitant thyroid pathology on preoperative workup for primary hyperparathyroidism. Eur J Med Res 2009; 14(1):37–41.
56. Abboud B, Sleilaty G, Rabaa L, et al. Ultrasonography: highly accuracy technique for preoperative localization of parathyroid adenoma. Laryngoscope 2008;118(9):1574–8.
57. Mazzeo S, Caramella D, Lencioni R, et al. Usefulness of echo-color Doppler in differentiating parathyroid lesions from other cervical masses. Eur Radiol 1997; 7(1):90–5.
58. Ahuja A, Ying M, King A, et al. Lymph node hilus: gray scale and power Doppler sonography of cervical nodes. J Ultrasound Med 2001;20:987–92.
59. Solorzano CC, Carneiro-Pla DM, Irvin GL. Surgeon-performed ultrasonography as the initial and only localizing study in sporadic primary hyperparathyroidism. J Am Coll Surg 2006;202(1):18–24.
60. Koslin DB, Adams J, Andersen P, et al. Preoperative evaluation of patients with primary hyperparathyroidism: role of high-resolution ultrasound. Laryngoscope 1997;107(9):1249–53.
61. Livingston CD, Victor B, Askew R, et al. Surgeon-performed ultrasonography as an adjunct to minimally invasive radio-guided parathyroidectomy in 100 consecutive patients with primary hyperparathyroidism. Endocr Pract 2008;14(1):28–32.
62. Stephen AE, Milas M, Garner CN, et al. Use of surgeon-performed office ultrasound and parathyroid fine needle aspiration for complex parathyroid localization. Surgery 2005;138(6):1143–50.
63. Veldman MW, Reading CC, Farrell MA, et al. Percutaneous parathyroid ethanol ablation in patients with multiple endocrine neoplasia type 1. AJR Am J Roentgenol 2008;191(6):1740–4.

Ultrasound-Guided Procedures for the Office

Russell B. Smith, MD[a,b,*]

KEYWORDS

- Ultrasound-guided • Fine-needle aspiration biopsy
- Interventional ultrasonography

Over the past decade, ultrasonography (US) has become an instrumental component in the diagnostic evaluation of a multitude of head and neck pathologies. The technology can also be beneficial for image guidance during percutaneous and open head and neck procedures. Although US-guided fine-needle aspiration biopsy (FNAB) accounts for the vast majority of these procedures, US guidance can also be used for aspiration of fluid collections and therapeutic injections as well as an intraoperative adjuvant to guide revision surgery. A thorough understanding of the capabilities of interventional US allows optimal management of a wide variety of complex clinical scenarios.

FINE-NEEDLE ASPIRATION BIOPSY

Masses of the head and neck are frequently evaluated by FNAB to establish a diagnosis. Although some head and neck masses are easily palpable and hand-guided FNAB is feasible, many masses are indistinct or not palpable and image-guided FNAB is required. Additionally, it is not uncommon for a thyroid nodule or malignant adenopathy of the neck to be a complex mass with both solid and cystic components. In this situation, US guidance can decrease the chance of a nondiagnostic biopsy by ensuring that the solid component of the mass is sampled during the procedure. US-guided FNAB for nodular disease of the thyroid is the most commonly performed US-guided procedure, but salivary gland masses and cervical adenopathy as well as a wide variety of unusual neck masses may require image guidance for cytologic assessment. In addition to understanding the indications for biopsy and mastering the techniques of performing a US-guided biopsy, it is critical that otolaryngologists

[a] Department of Otolaryngology—Head and Neck Surgery, 981225 University of Nebraska Medical Center, Omaha, NE 68198, USA
[b] Nebraska Methodist Estabrook Cancer Center, Omaha, NE, USA
* Department of Otolaryngology—Head and Neck Surgery, 981225 University of Nebraska Medical Center, Omaha, NE 68198.
E-mail address: rbsmith@unmc.edu

Otolaryngol Clin N Am 43 (2010) 1241–1254
doi:10.1016/j.otc.2010.08.007
0030-6665/10/$ – see front matter © 2010 Elsevier Inc. All rights reserved.

possess a thorough understanding of the limitations and potential pitfalls of FNAB in the assessment of masses in these areas.

Thyroid

In patients with thyroid nodules, many factors are considered when determining whether or not surgical intervention is required. Because most thyroid nodules are asymptomatic and nonfunctional, the key determinant of the need for surgery is the risk that a nodule represents a neoplasm. Although history, physical examination, and specific US features can assist otolaryngologists in determining the potential for neoplasm, FNAB is considered the most accurate diagnostic evaluation to assess for malignancy (**Fig. 1**). In patients with larger nodules, palpation-guided FNAB can be easily performed in the outpatient setting without the need for image guidance. But, many thyroid nodules are not easily palpable and image guidance is required to complete the biopsy. Additionally, some palpable thyroid nodules can be complex masses with dominant cystic components. In this scenario, US guidance to ensure sampling of the solid component is valuable to ensure a diagnostic biopsy. Comparisons of palpation-guided and US-guided FNAB for thyroid nodules suggest that US-guided FNAB is more accurate and results in a lower rate of nondiagnostic

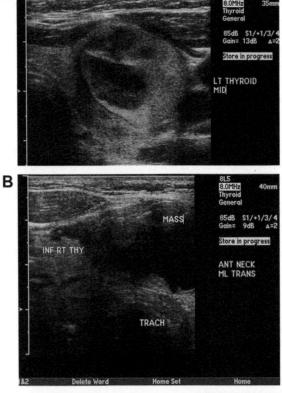

Fig. 1. US of thyroid nodules. Distinctly different-appearing thyroid nodules by US. (A) Thyroid nodule with US features suggestive of a benign nodule. (B) Thyroid nodule with US features suggestive of malignancy. Final histopathologic evaluation revealed both nodules to be follicular thyroid cancer.

biopsies. In a review of 376 FNABs of the thyroid, Izquierdo and colleagues[1] reported that for palpable thyroid nodules, US-guided FNAB was 20% more accurate (80%) and had a lower incidence of nondiagnostic specimens (7.1%) when compared with palpation-guided FNAB.

Recently, the National Cancer Institute proposed a 6-tiered classification scheme for the assessment of thyroid FNAB (**Table 1**).[2] Based on this system, the risk of malignancy for a thyroid nodule is defined and guidelines for management are proposed. In patients with nodules that by FNAB are suggestive of neoplasm, suspicious for malignancy, or malignant, surgery is recommended.[3] It is critical, however, to consider FNAB as only one component of the diagnostic evaluation of a patient with a thyroid nodule. In patients with history, physical examination, or imaging findings suggestive of malignancy, surgery should be recommended even if the FNAB is interpreted as low risk of malignancy.

In addition to the cytologic assessment of FNAB in a patient with suspected well-differentiated thyroid cancer, assessment for thyroglobulin in the saline washout of the needle after biopsy of a mass can be performed. Especially if a mass is suspected to be recurrent disease and has negative cytology, this technique can be a useful method to confirm the presence of disease. This technique can be used on masses suspected to be local or nodal recurrences, with the greatest benefit in lesions smaller than 1 cm.[4] After a 1-mL saline washout, a thyroglobulin of greater than 4 to 10 ng/mL has been established as indicative of disease, but false-positive results can occur.[4–6] This technique is valid even in patients who have antithyroglobulin antibodies.[7] Analysis for BRAF can also be completed on material obtained by FNAB in patients suspected of having papillary thyroid cancer. In the future, such an assessment may be important in surgical planning because patients with BRAF mutations are known to have more aggressive disease.[8]

In a fashion similar to thyroglobulin washout in patients with well-differentiated thyroid cancer, calcitonin washout can be performed in patients suspected of having primary or recurrent medullary thyroid cancer. In 36 patients suspected of having medullary thyroid cancer, the sensitivity and specificity of calcitonin washout has been reported as 100%, with FNAB cytologic evaluation having a sensitivity of 62% and specificity of 80%.[9] Although a calcitonin greater than 36 pg/mL is indicative of medullary thyroid cancer, others have found that patients with benign thyroid conditions can have calcitonin washout as high as 67 pg/mL and that in cases of medullary thyroid cancer the calcitonin washout was extremely high.[9,10]

Table 1		
National Cancer Institute thyroid FNAB guidelines committee IV		
Suggested Category	**Alternate Category**	**Risk of Malignancy**
Benign		<1%
Atypia of undetermined significance	Indeterminant follicular lesions rule out neoplasm Atypical follicular lesion Cellular follicular lesion	5%–10%
Neoplasm	Suspicious for neoplasms	20%–30%
Suspicious for malignancy		50%–75%
Malignant		100%
Nondiagnostic	Unsatisfactory	—

Parathyroid

Unlike nodular disease of the thyroid, which routinely undergoes cytologic assessment, rarely is it necessary to perform FNAB for parathyroid pathology. For patients with hyperparathyroidism, the need for surgery is based on the metabolic sequelae of the disease rather than the concern that the disease represents malignancy. The success of parathyroidectomy for hyperparathyroidism is high with cure rates greater than 95%, obviating FNAB to confirm suspected lesions as parathyroid in origin.

In the small subset of patients who have persistent or recurrent hyperparathyroidism after prior surgical explorations, FNAB can play a role in the localization of the disease. In cases of persistent/recurrent disease, the pathology is usually located in the previously dissected central compartment. Subsequently, use of FNAB to confirm that suspicious lesions in previously operated fields are of parathyroid origin can be beneficial before revision surgery. When performing FNAB to confirm parathyroid disease, consider obtaining a parathyroid hormone washout of the aspirate in addition to cytologic assessment. Agrawal and colleagues reported limitations with cytologic evaluation of suspected parathyroid lesions by FNAB. In their series of 53 patients undergoing FNAB of suspected parathyroid lesions, the cytologic evaluation was able to identify parathyroid cells in only 40% of aspirates, with 28% of the aspirated being nondiagnostic.[11] Although the features of monomorphic cells with stippled nuclear chromatin in the absence of atypia, mitosis, or prominent nucleoli are suggestive of parathyroid origin, distinguishing parathyroid from thyroid tissue can be problematic especially if there is not any colloid in the specimen. Erbil and colleagues assessed the role of parathyroid hormone washout on the FNAB of lesions of the central compartment. Lesions suspected of parathyroid origin could be consistently discriminated from thyroid pathology with the parathyroid lesions having an average parathyroid hormone level of 4700 pg/mL compared to 48 pg/mL in the thyroid lesions.[12]

Salivary Gland

A wide variety of benign and malignant neoplasms can affect the major and minor salivary glands. Additionally, some non-neoplastic diseases can present as a salivary gland mass. The vast majority of salivary gland neoplasms are located in the parotid gland. The use of FNAB for salivary gland neoplasms is controversial, but it should be considered in the diagnostic evaluation of a patient with a salivary gland mass. Opponents of FNAB of salivary gland neoplasms feel that surgical excision should be performed for all tumors and that cytologic diagnosis does not significantly alter the treatment plan. Proponents of FNAB of salivary gland neoplasms feel that cytologic information assists in determining the risk of malignancy, allowing for optimal surgical planning and patient counseling preoperatively.

Given the wide variety of benign neoplasms as well as low-grade and high-grade malignancies that can affect the salivary glands, limitations exist regarding the ability of FNAB to establish a definitive diagnosis. Although some benign neoplasms, such as pleomorphic adenoma and Warthin tumor, can be accurately diagnosed by FNAB, other pathologies are more difficult to specifically classify on FNAB. For example, differentiating a cellular pleomorphic adenoma from a low-grade basal cell adenocarcinoma cannot be accomplished. Additionally, determining the exact pathologic subtype of a high-grade carcinoma is not possible (**Table 2**). The ability of US-guided FNAB of salivary gland neoplasms to distinguish benign from malignant tumors is high, with Bajaj and colleagues[13] reporting a sensitivity of 85%, specificity of 96%, and overall accuracy of 94%. Others have proposed core biopsy as the preferred technique for assessment of salivary gland neoplasms. Buckland and colleagues[14]

Table 2
Erroneous diagnoses of fine-needle aspiration biopsy of salivary gland masses

Erroneous FNAB Result	Actual Diagnosis
Benign lymphoid tissue	Acinic cell carcinoma
	Lymphoma
	Warthin tumor
Non-neoplastic gland	Acinic cell carcinoma
	Pleomorphic adenoma
	Squamous cell carcinoma, mucoepidermoid carcinoma
	Warthin tumor
Pleomorphic adenoma	Adenoid cystic carcinoma
Basal cell adenoma	Basal cell adenocarcinoma
	Adenoid cystic carcinoma
Adenoid cystic carcinoma	Pleomorphic adenoma
	Basal cell adenoma

reported 100% accuracy for US-guided core biopsy, with nearly all the masses in the series having undergone a prior FNAB that was nondiagnostic. The slightly more invasive nature of a core biopsy must be considered before implementing routine use of this technique. Overall, there is little doubt that FNAB can play a vital role in the assessment of select patients with a salivary gland mass.

Lymph Node

Although a lateral neck mass may represent a wide variety of pathology, it is frequently the result of an enlarged lymph node. In patients with cervical lymphadenopathy, infectious, inflammatory, and neoplastic diagnoses must be considered. A patient's age, recent health status, history of exposure to carcinogens, and clinical characteristics of the mass are important factors in determining the probability that a neck mass may be malignant. FNAB is frequently performed on cervical lymphadenopathy to assess for malignancy before surgical excision of the mass. If possible, the surgeon should avoid the clinical scenario of performing an excisional biopsy of a lymph node and being surprised by the final pathology revealing carcinoma.

As with thyroid, parathyroid, and salivary gland pathology, US guidance for FNAB of cervical lymphadenopathy offers significant benefit. For malignant adenopathy, significant necrosis can be present and US guidance to the more solid areas of the lymph node can produce a higher yield of diagnostic biopsies. Conversely, in patients with presumed cervical lymphadenitis, US guidance can be used to access small areas of suppuration within the node to obtain a specimen for gram stain and cultures. Even in cases of suspected benign disease resulting in cervical lymphadenopathy, biopsy may play a role in establishing a diagnosis. Kim and colleagues reported on the use of US-guided core biopsies of cervical adenopathy in patients without known malignancy. Diagnostic specimens were obtained in 94% with a reported accuracy of 98% based on histologic confirmation of excisional biopsies or regression of suspected benign lesions.[15] The histologic diagnoses included reactive hyperplasia in 44 patients, tuberculosis in 37 patients, Kikuchi disease in 25 patients, metastasis in 16 patients, lymphoma in 16 patients, normal in 7 patients, and toxoplasmosis in 1 patient.

DRAINAGE PROCEDURES

Fluid collections are frequently encountered in the head and neck region. These collections may be the consequence of an infection with abscess formation, hemorrhage into an existing cyst, or a postoperative complication. US-guided drainage may be an appropriate intervention, depending on the clinical scenario, and allow an otolaryngologist to avoid an open surgical procedure for the management of the disease (**Fig. 2**). Chang and colleagues reported successful management of deep neck abscesses in 14 patients using US-guided drainage. Especially in patients with well-defined, unilocular abscesses, US drainage with or without drain placement should be considered without concern of complicating a future open drainage procedure if required.[16]

INJECTION PROCEDURES

Although injection procedures are the least commonly performed application of interventional US in the head and neck, it can be extremely valuable for certain clinical scenarios. These interventions may be for the injection of ablative or sclerosing agents

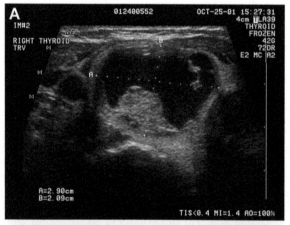

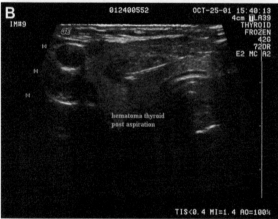

Fig. 2. US guidance for drainage of a thyroid hematoma. Patient presenting with an acutely enlarging mass in the thyroid. (*A*) US shows a complex-appearing mass with a large anechoic component. This was an intrathyroidal hematoma as a result of a neck trauma (strangulation). (*B*) US shows needle localized in area with near-total decompression of the hematoma. (*Courtesy of* Dr Robert Sofferman, MD.)

or botulinum toxin A as well as placement of localization guide wires to assist with surgical resection (**Fig. 3**). Although these procedures can be safely performed, ensuring that the injection is not accidentally placed into a vascular structure is critical.

Success has been reported with the use of 95% ethanol for ablation of lesions in the head and neck, especially in those who are at high risk of undergoing surgical resection because of poor medical status or concerns of surgical morbidity due to prior therapy. This approach has been successfully performed for autonomous thyroid nodules, recurrent well-differentiated thyroid cancer, and recurrent primary hyperparathyroidism.[17–19] Some discomfort should be expected with these procedures and liberal application of local anesthetic in the skin as well as deeply around the area to be ablated should be performed. Temporary nerve paralysis has been reported with this technique.[19]

In patients with cerebral palsy, sialorrhea can be a major issue that negatively affects the quality of life of the patients as well as their caregivers.[20] Sialorrhea can also be a major issue in adults who have degenerative neurologic diseases, such as Parkinson disease and amyotrophic lateral sclerosis.[21,22] For these conditions, intraglandular injection of botulinum toxin A can be effective in managing sialorrhea without a negative impact on the adjacent musculature. For these cases, US guidance to localize the needle within the parenchyma of the submandibular and the parotid glands can be used to ensure appropriate placement of the botulinum toxin A injection.

TECHNICAL CONSIDERATIONS IN INTERVENTIONAL ULTRASONOGRAPHY

To optimize the success of US-guided procedures, one must ensure that the patient is comfortably positioned and that the required supplies are available in the procedural suite. Developing a protocol/checklist for the staff assisting with the procedure can greatly facilitate this process. In addition to preparing the procedural room, the staff can assist with the procedure by manipulating the aspiration syringe as well as performing video documentation during the biopsy. Finally, communication with the

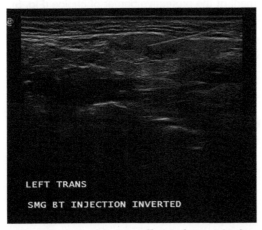

Fig. 3. Injection procedure. Patient with ALS suffering from sialorrhea. The US shows the needle with tip in submandibular gland. The hypoechoic changes noted at the tip of the needle is a result of the botulinum toxin A injection infiltrating the parenchyma of the gland. (*Courtesy of* Dr Lisa Orloff, MD.)

Pathology department is critical to ensure that the biopsy specimen is prepared using methods that meet the needs of the cytologist.

Patient Preparation

Ensuring that the patient is comfortable for the procedure is critical to the success of US-guided interventions. If a patient is experiencing pain at the site of needle placement or is positioned such that the head and neck are not adequately supported, movement inevitably will occur. Any movement complicates needle placement and potentially decreases the success of the procedure.

Infiltration of the skin and subcutaneous tissues with local anesthetic should be completed before the procedure. An area approximately 2 cm in diameter should be anesthetized. The most efficient method to accurately place the local anesthetic is to put the patient in the identical position planned for the procedure. After positioning has been complete, US should be performed to localize the area of interest. Once the area of interest is well visualized with the probe positioned on the neck in the same fashion as it would be for the biopsy, the site at which the biopsy needle will enter the skin can be marked (**Fig. 4**). The local anesthetic can then be infiltrated around the area identified as the biopsy site. Additional local anesthetic can be placed along the planned needle path to the area to be biopsied if desired, but this is not frequently required.

Equipment and Supplies

As with diagnostic US of the head and neck, high-resolution US (8–12 MHz) should be used when performing image-guided procedures. Most commonly, a linear transducer is used during the procedure. It is important to optimize the setting of the US equipment based on the location and size of the mass to be biopsied. Ensure that the image contrast, magnification, and focal area are appropriately set before the procedure. The transducer must be prepared for the procedure to ensure that it is not exposed to body fluids or alcohol, which is used as asepsis for the skin. Several commercially available US probe covers are available, but cling wrap is a cost-effective alternative. A generous amount of US gel should be placed on the end of the transducer before placement of the protective barrier of choice (**Fig. 5**).

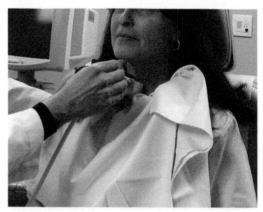

Fig. 4. Patient marking for local anesthetic infiltration. Once the US probe is localized in a position similar to that to be used for biopsy, the skin can be marked at the site at which the needle will be entered into the skin.

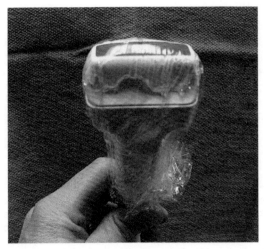

Fig. 5. Preparation of the US probe for needle biopsy. The US probe has US gel applied followed by coverage with a cling wrap before biopsy.

A multitude of supplies are required to perform percutaneous procedures in the head and neck (**Box 1**). Although alcohol preparation of the skin is adequate, Betadine or other sterile prep solutions can be considered per operator preference. Glass slides with fixative, Cytolye solution, and sterile containers for cultures should be prepared depending on the procedure being completed. Adhesive bandage and ice packs also need to be available for postprocedure care of the patient (**Fig. 6**).

The vast majority of FNAB are performed with either a 22Ga or a 25Ga needle. For drainage procedures, at least a 20Ga and preferably an 18Ga needle are used. The needle for injection procedures is typically a 25Ga needle, but if injecting a more viscous material, a larger needle may be required. A needle length of 1.5 in is adequate

Box 1
Supplies for interventional ultrasonography
Alcohol prep pad
Skin marking pin
Syringe for local anesthetic
Syringe for aspiration
Needles (18, 22, 25, 27 Ga)
Local anesthetic
Intravenous tubing—optional
Needle aspiration gun—optional
Slides and fixative for smear preparation of the biopsy
CytoLyt for preparation of cell block
Adhesive bandage
Ice pack

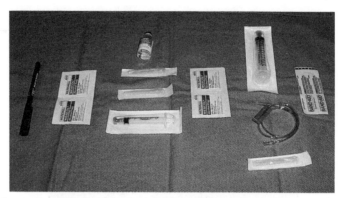

Fig. 6. Basic supplies used for office-based US procedures. Skin marker to mark site of local anesthetic infiltration; small syringe (3–5 μL) with needles for administration of local anesthetic; alcohol for skin prep before placement of anesthetic as well as biopsy; syringe and intravenous tubing; needle for biopsy; and adhesive bandage for biopsy site post procedure.

for the vast majority of lesions, but longer needles may be required for deep lesions or those that require a greater angle of approach to access the lesion. For fine-needle aspiration and drainage procedures, the needle may be directly attached to the syringe or an 8- to 12-in intravenous tubing may be used between the needle and the syringe. The advantage of using intravenous tubing is that it allows the assistant to manipulate the syringe for aspiration while the surgeon can focus efforts on needle localization and movement within the area of interest depending on the procedure performed. For injection procedures, it is best to have the needle directly attached to the syringe to avoid waste of the injection material within the intravenous tubing.

Performing the Procedure

When performing US-guided procedures, two approaches can be used for needle placement. The approach used is predominantly influenced by the preference of the otolaryngologist performing the biopsy. In certain situations, one approach may be preferred due to anatomic considerations of the area of interest. The difference in the techniques is based on the relationship of the needle to the US transducer. The long-axis technique involves introducing the needle into the skin along the narrow side of transducer with the needle advanced parallel to area imaged (**Fig. 7**). With the short-axis technique, the needle is placed in the skin along the long side of the transducer and then advanced obliquely across the area imaged (**Fig. 8**).

Although the long-axis technique requires a slightly longer pathway to the area of interest, it has the advantage of allowing visualization of the entire needle during the procedure (**Fig. 9**). When using the long-axis technique, lesions that are deeply seated between anatomic structures may require that the US probe is oriented in the saggital plane instead of the axial plane when performing the biopsy. An example is a deeply located thyroid nodule positioned in between the trachea and carotid artery.

With the short-axis technique, a shorter needle pathway is used and almost every procedure can be performed while using axial imaging of the neck. The technique requires that the operator is comfortable seeing only the tip of the needle during the procedure instead of the entire needle (**Fig. 10**).

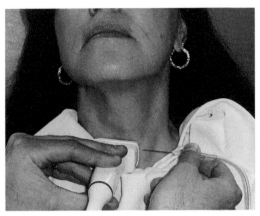

Fig. 7. Long-axis technique of needle placement. The needle is placed along the narrow side of transducer and advanced parallel to the imaged area.

Considerations for Fine-Needle Aspiration Biopsy

Prior to inserting the needle into the area of interest, the plunger should be drawn back to allow at least 2 to 3 mL of air into the chamber. Once the needle is accurately placed into the mass of interest, slight negative pressure can be applied to the syringe and the needle is then moved rhythmically within the mass. Although sampling different areas of a mass should be considered, it is recommended that, with each biopsy, the needle passes focus on a small region and that each pass of the needle not randomly move to a different area of the mass.

With subsequent biopsies, a similar technique can be performed on different areas within the mass. The number of needle passes recommended varies and can be as few as 2 to 3 passes and up to as many as 10 passes with each needle placement. Additional passes can be considered if no material is seen accumulating in the hub of the needle. Additionally, if a brisk return of blood or fluid is obtained, the number of needle passes in that area should be limited and the needle relocated to a different area of the mass. It must be ensured that the assistant has released all the negative

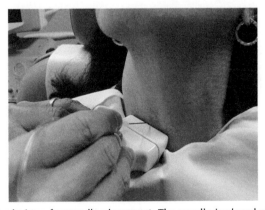

Fig. 8. Short-axis technique for needle placement. The needle is placed along the long side of transducer and advanced obliquely to the imaged area.

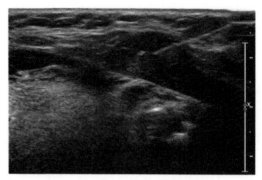

Fig. 9. US of long-axis technique. The entire needle path can be seen with the tip of the needle in the area to be biopsied.

pressure off the syringe before removing the needle from the area biopsied to avoid contaminants being drawn into the needle as well as to prevent the aspirate from being drawn all the way into the chamber of the syringe on exit of the skin.

Typically, three separate needle sampling are performed for each mass. Biopsy using a capillary technique has also been successful for cytologic assessment of a mass.[23] With this approach, a syringe is still needed to expel the biopsy material onto the slides once the biopsy has been completed.

Considerations for Drainage

A similar approach to FNAB may be used for drainage procedures. In this situation, the use of intravenous tubing has the advantages of allowing a surgeon to more freely move the needle to areas requiring drainage during the procedure while an assistant maintains negative pressure on the syringe. The use of intravenous tubing also allows the assistant to easily switch the syringe when filled so that the drainage procedure can be continued without having to remove the needle.

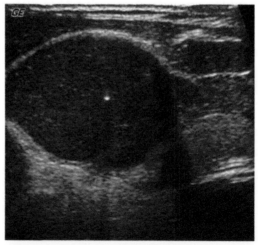

Fig. 10. US of short-axis technique. The tip of the needle is seen in the middle of the area of interest.

During the procedure, the surgeon should visualize the evacuation of the fluid collection. This allows the surgeon to move the needle to areas of residual fluid, which may be due to loculations or gravity-dependent areas in the neck. For larger fluid collections, external manipulation of the soft tissue of neck can be performed by the assistant to direct residual fluid toward the needle to facilitate evacuation of the area. Percutaneous drain placement can be considered as part of the procedure based on the management requirements of the disease.

Injection

Injection of therapeutic agents using US guidance ensures delivery of the agent to the target area and not into adjacent critical structures. For most procedures, a volume of less than 1 mL is used. Injection of small volumes helps ensure that limited to no extravasation of the injected agent occurs. For botulinum toxin A injections, each gland receives two intraglandular injections with a total dose of 125 U required.[21] For ethanol ablative therapy, a total volume of 0.5 to 1 mL is injected as multiple 0.1-mL aliquots throughout the mass. With ethanol therapy, the area injected quickly becomes intensely echogenic. This lasts approximately 1 minute and should be allowed to resolve before attempting additional injections to ensure that the needle tip is not obscured.[18,19] Other agents may also be used depending on the clinical scenario and the specific characteristics of each agent must be understood to allow safe injection.

CONCLUSION: APPLICATIONS FOR INTERVENTIONAL ULTRASOUND OF HEAD AND NECK

There are many applications for interventional US in the head and neck. Although FNAB is the most common performed image-guided procedure, a host of other interventions can be of clinical benefit. The success of US-guided procedures is dependent on many factors, but the technique can be easily mastered by otolaryngologists.

REFERENCES

1. Izquierdo R, Arekat MR, Knudson PE, et al. Comparison of palpation-guided and ultrasound-guided fine-needle biopsies of thyroid nodules in an outpatient endocrinology practice. Endocr Pract 2006;12:609–14.
2. Baloch ZW, Ciabs ES, Clak DP, et al. The National Cancer Institute thyroid fine needle aspiration state of the science conference: a summation. Cytojournal 2008;5:6.
3. Layfield LJ, Cibas ES, Gharib H, et al. Thyroid aspiration cytology: current status. CA Cancer J Clin 2009;59:99–110.
4. Lee YH, Seo HS, Suh SI, et al. Cut-off value for needle washout thyroglobulin in athyrotropic patients. Laryngoscope 2010;120:1120–4.
5. Mikosiriski S, Pomorski L, Oszukowska L, et al. The diagnostic value of thyroglobulin concentration in fine-needle aspiration of the cervical lymph nodes in patients with differentiated thyroid cancer. Endorkrynol Pol 2006;57:392–5.
6. Kim MJ, Kim EK, Kim BM, et al. Thyroglobulin measurement in fine-needle aspiration washouts: the criteria for neck node dissection for patients with thyroid cancer. Clin Endocrinol (Oxf) 2009;70:145–51.
7. Boi F, Baghino G, Atzeni F, et al. The diagnostic value for differentiated thyroid carcinoma metastases of thyroglobulin (Tg) measurement in washout fluid from fine-needle aspiration biopsy of neck lymph nodes is maintained in the presence of circulating anti-Tg antibodies. J Clin Endocrinol Metab 2006;91:1364–9.

8. Xing M. BRAF mutation in thyroid cancer. Endocr Relat Cancer 2005;12:245–62.

9. Boi F, Maurelli I, Pinna G, et al. Calcitonin measurement in wash-out fluid from fine needle aspiration of neck masses in patients with primary and metastatic medullary thyroid carcinoma. Clin Endocrinol Metab 2007;92:2115–8.

10. Kudo T, Miyauchi A, Ito Y, et al. Diagnosis of medullary thyroid carcinoma by calcitonin measurement in fine-needle aspiration biopsy specimens. Thyroid 2007;17:635–8.

11. Agarwal AM, Bentz JS, Hungerford R, et al. Parathyroid fine-needle aspiration cytology in the evaluation of parathyroid adenoma: cytologic findings from 53 patients. Diagn Cytopathol 2009;37:407–10.

12. Erbil Y, Barbaros U, Salmaslioglu A, et al. Value o13.f parathyroid hormone assay for preoperative sonographically guided parathyroid aspirates for minimally invasive parathyroidectomy. J Clin Ultrasound 2006;34:425–9.

13. Bajaj Y, Singh S, Cozens N, et al. Critical clinical appraisal of the role of ultrasound guided fine needle aspiration cytology in the management of parotid tumors. J Laryngol Otol 2005;119:289–92.

14. Buckland JR, Manjaly G, Violaris N, et al. Ultrasound-guided cutting needle biopsy of the parotid gland. J Laryngol Otol 1999;113:988–92.

15. Kim BM, Kim EK, Kim MJ, et al. Sonographically guided core needle biopsy of cervical lymphadenopathy in patients without known malignancy. J Ultrasound Med 2007;26:585–91.

16. Chang KP, Chen YL, Hao SP, et al. Ultrasound-guided closed drainage for abscesses of the head and neck. Otolaryngol Head Neck Surg 2005;132:119–24.

17. Golletti O, Monzani F, Caraccio N, et al. Percutaneous ethanol injection treatment of autonomously functioning single thyroid nodules: optimization of treatment and short term outcome. World J Surg 1992;16:784–9.

18. Lewis BD, Hay ID, Charboneau JW, et al. Percutaneous ethanol injection for treatment of cervical lymph node metastases in patients with papillary thyroid carcinoma. Am J Roentgenol 2002;178:699–704.

19. Harman CR, Grant CS, Hay ID, et al. Indications, technique, and efficacy of alcohol injection of enlarged parathyroid glands in patients with primary hyperparathyroidism. Surgery 1998;124:1011–20.

20. Banerjee KJ, Glasson C, O'Flaherty SJ. Parotid and submandibular botulinum toxin A injections for sialorrhea in children with cerebral palsy. Dev Med Child Neurol 2006;48:883–7.

21. Nobrega AC, Rodrigues B, Melo A. Does botulinum toxin injection in parotid glands interfere with the swallowing dynamics of Parkinson's disease patients? Clin Neurol Neurosurg 2009;111:430–2.

22. Gilio F, Iacovelli E, Frasca V, et al. Botulinum toxin type A for treatment of sialorrhea in amyotropic lateral sclerosis: a clinical and neurophysiologic study. Amyotroph Lateral Scler 2010;11:359–63.

23. De Carvalho GA, Paz-Filho G, Cavalcanti TC, et al. Adequacy and diagnostic accuracy of aspiration vs. capillary fine needle thyroid biopsies. Endocr Pathol 2009;20:204–8.

Head and Neck Ultrasound in the Pediatric Population

Veronica J. Rooks, MD[a,b], Benjamin B. Cable, MD[a,c],*

KEYWORDS

- Pediatric • Head and neck ultrasound • Otolaryngology
- Office imaging

ADVANTAGES OF OFFICE IMAGING STUDIES OF THE HEAD AND NECK IN CHILDREN

Diagnostic imaging studies of the head and neck in children have three main challenges. First, pediatric conditions that require imaging are often dynamic and changing. Examples include lymphadenopathy, deep neck space infections, and vascular malformations. Although an initial imaging study can offer a great deal of information, it remains a snapshot in time and does not offer the physician insight beyond a narrow period. Many pediatric lesions quickly evolve over days or weeks, making remote imaging less relevant. Also, virtually all pediatric imaging is done outside the otolaryngology clinic. This not only requires additional logistics but also is accompanied by an interruption in care. In most major medical centers, imaging is scheduled hours, days, or weeks after the initial clinic visit. Once completed, the study must be conveyed back to the managing provider for review and decision making. Finally, many pediatric imaging studies require sedation or even general anesthesia for adequate information to be gained. This adds further logistical challenges to the health care team and poses additional risk to the patient.

In selected cases, directed ultrasound has the potential to solve all three of these major issues. Ultrasound devices are now portable enough to be brought directly to the operating room, clinic examination room, or bedside and can be used by a radiologist or otolaryngologist with little preparation. Examinations are usually completed in minutes, can frequently be performed during the initial consultation, and are well tolerated in most children. With no need for radiation exposure, intravenous medication, or

The authors have no financial disclosures.

[a] Uniformed Services University of the Health Sciences, Bethesda, MD, USA

[b] Pediatric Radiology, Department of Radiology, Tripler Army Medical Center, 1 Jarrett White Road, TAMC, Honolulu, HI 96859, USA

[c] Pediatric Otolaryngology/Head & Neck Surgery, Tripler Army Medical Center, 3C ENT Clinic, 1 Jarrett White Road, Honolulu, TAMC, HI 96859, USA

* Corresponding author. Pediatric Otolaryngology/Head & Neck Surgery, Tripler Army Medical Center, 3C ENT Clinic, 1 Jarrett White Road, Honolulu, TAMC, HI 96859.

E-mail address: benjamin.cable@us.army.mil

sedation, it can be repeated as often as needed rather than offering a single snap-shot of the lesion in question; ultrasound can be repeatedly used to track the evolution of lesions before, sometimes during, and after treatment.

Pediatric head and neck ultrasound uses the same hardware used in adult applications. No additional supplies are needed. Machines range in size from moderate-sized carts to laptop versions that are placed on wheeled stands. Each of the machines fit into a standard size examination room and, with battery backup, can be moved between treatment areas without interruption. Image storage varies between machines and ranges across the standard data formats and, depending on hospital archive systems, may or may not be available throughout the hospital. Although many probe types exist, a single high-frequency linear probe, 8 to 15 MHz, is adequate for most applications in otolaryngology. Specific courses in pediatric ultrasound for otolaryngologists do not yet exist. Despite this lack, current course offerings dealing with adult ultrasound are offered to otolaryngologists through the American College of Surgeons. Techniques reviewed and evaluated at these training events are highly relevant to pediatric applications. Along with outside training, partnership with one's own radiology team is indispensable for advice and training as comfort is gained with the basic examination and techniques.

SPECIFIC APPLICATIONS OF ULTRASOUND IN THE OTOLARNGOLOGY CLINIC
Lymphadenopathy

Evaluation of lymphadenopathy in children can quickly be accomplished with ultrasound. In the authors' clinic, ultrasound has evolved to become a natural extension of the physical examination. Although palpation of lymphadenopathy in most children is simple, accurate sizing of lymph nodes and diagnosis of multiple contiguous nodes is often difficult. Overlying tissue frequently adds to the perceived size of the lymph nodes. Ultrasound offers solutions to both problems. With a brief imaging examination done to enhance palpation, the location of the lymphadenopathy is quickly determined. Precise sizing can be performed with digital calipers. Specific nodal architecture can often be visualized. Normal or reactive lymph nodes should typically be well defined and elliptical in shape. Their parenchyma should be homogeneously hypoechoic with a central linear-hyperechoic vascular hilum (**Fig. 1**). Although no ultrasound findings have been strongly correlated with neoplasm, concerns for malignancy arise with loss of the normal architecture, loss of the kidney bean shape to a more bulbous or round shape, absent hilum, irregular borders, cystic necrosis, and irregular capsular vasculature.[1] With baseline data established during initial consultation, children can be monitored with serial ultrasound examinations while undergoing medical evaluation and treatment. Any nodes that remain enlarged or demonstrate multiple abnormal findings despite treatment can be documented and targeted for excisional biopsy as indicated.

Branchial Cleft Anomalies and Thyroglossal Duct Cysts

Ultrasound can be used to evaluate branchial cleft anomalies and thyroglossal duct cysts (**Figs. 2** and **3**). In each case, cysts often present as thin-walled ovoid or round masses with significant heterogeneity and a lack of vascular architecture. Because 90% of branchial cleft cysts have origins in the second arch, most are frequently confirmed to be anterior to the sternocleidomastoid whereas thyroglossal duct cysts are most frequently localized within or in close proximity to the strap musculature.[2] Thyroglossal duct cysts can, in rare circumstances, represent ectopic thyroid tissue. Confirmation of normal thyroid architecture below the mass in question is recommended before surgery is undertaken.[3] Ultrasound can easily accomplish this task during the same examination done for mass evaluation.

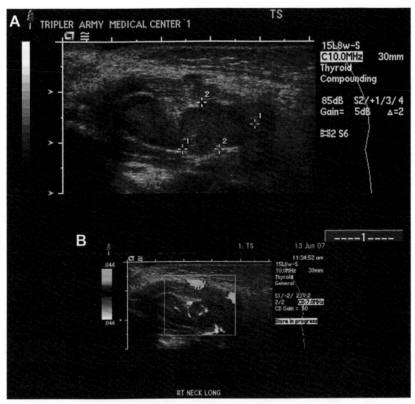

Fig. 1. (*A*) Five-month-old with fevers to 103°F for 36 hours with increased swelling of right neck. Screening ultrasound images demonstrate bilobed solid structures with hypoechoic peripheral parenchyma and central increased hilar echogenicity, consistent with a reactive lymph node. (*B*) Central color Doppler flow is noted, characteristic for a lymph node. Electronic calipers allow incremental follow-up to the scale of a millimeter.

Vascular and Lymphatic Malformations

Vascular and lymphatic malformations are both amenable to ultrasound evaluation. Although various classification schemes exist, mixed lesions are possible and, in the authors' opinion, more frequent than often reported. Purely lymphatic malformations are often encountered in the posterior cervical space and within the oral cavity. Ultrasound examination demonstrates cysts with variable thickness to their septa and heterogeneous fluid levels within (**Fig. 4**).[2] Ultrasound examination can rapidly define microcystic disease from macrocystic elements. Doppler color flow examination is invaluable in this setting and quickly confirms lack of significant blood flow. Finding significant random blood flow patterns within a lesion provides evidence for a vascular or mixed lesion (**Fig. 5**). Flow rates within these lesions can be subjectively observed and low-flow versus high-flow status can be seen in real time.

Abscesses

Ultrasound can be used to evaluate possible abscess formation. Classically, deep neck space infections have been limited to expansion within potential spaces and limited by fascial planes. With the advent of methicillin-resistant *Staphylococcus*

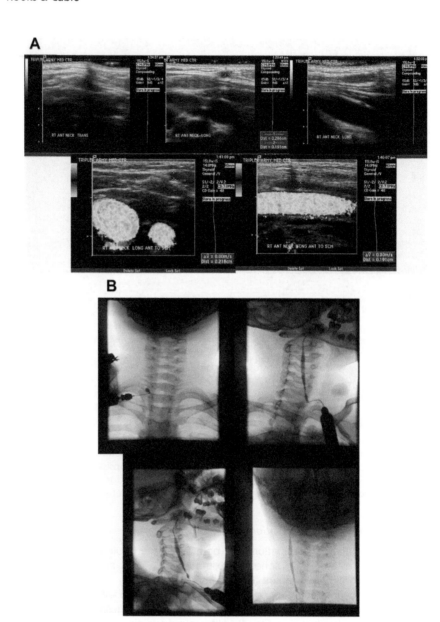

Fig. 2. (A) Five-year-old's complaint of "orange juice comes out this hole in my neck." Thyroglossal duct fistula ultrasound images demonstrate transverse and longitudinal images of the hypoechoic tract extending from skin surface, heading superiorly along carotid artery. (B) Fluoroscopic spot images after catheritization with angiocatheter and injection of contrast media demonstrate fistula tract from skin surface to pyriform sinus, consistent with branchial cleft fistula.

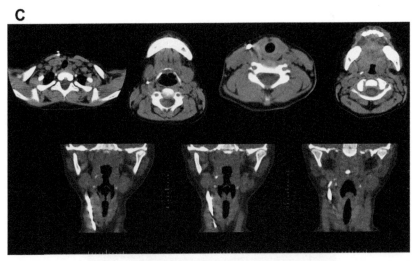

Fig. 2. (*C*) Axial and coronal reformatted images demonstrate skin orifice origin at the inferior-middle two-thirds junction of sternocleidomastoid muscle (SCM); deep to platysma; lateral to cranial nerves IX, X, and XII; between the internal and external carotid; and terminating in the tonsillar fossa.

aureus, otolaryngologists have begun to see more cases of superficial cellulitis lead to abscesss formation.[4,5] These superficial abcesesses with overlying cellulitis are often difficult to examine by palpation alone. Ultrasound again offers an augmentation of the physical examination in these situations and can quickly identify the border between soft tissue and the pus within an abscess cavity. Needle localization with or without excision and drainage can follow and total evacuation of the cavity can be confirmed.

Other Applications

Many other clinical applications for diagnostic ultrasound have been reported in the pediatric population. Infants born with an anterior neck mass and torticollis can be evaluated for pseudotumor of infancy with ultrasound alone (**Fig. 6**).[6] This modality can be used in the clinic to obviate CT or MRI evaluation. Laryngeal studies in children have been undertaken to assess dynamic vocal cord function and papilloma status in patients with known disease.[7,8] Thyroid mass evaluation can be performed in children as it is done in adults. Finally, ultrasonography has even been found to be an accurate method of confirming middle ear fluid and further defining the viscosity of the effusion.[9]

SPECIFIC APPLICATIONS IN THE OTOLARYNGOLOGY OPERATING ROOM
Intralesional Laser Treatment of Vascular Lesions

First introduced to the pediatric otolaryngology community by Brietzke and colleagues in 2001, intralesional laser treatment has become a viable tool for treating the spectrum of vascular lesions.[10] Using this technique, ultrasound evaluation is performed in a clinical setting and then confirmed at the time of surgery. Under ultrasound guidance, an 18-gauge intravenous catheter is introduced into the lesion and directed toward small to medium-sized feeding vasculature or central parenchyma (**Fig. 7**). Using a 600-μm fiber introduced through the intravenous catheter,

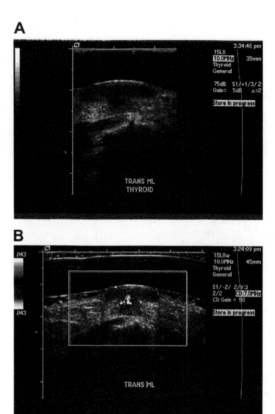

Fig. 3. (A) Thyroglossal duct cyst in a 10-year-old boy with midline cervical palpable mass. Transverse sonogram demonstrates an oval, well-defined, hypoechoic mass with through transmission in the suprahyoid neck midline. Note anechoic standoff pad placed between transducer and skin surface to facilitate superficial lesions. (B) Color Doppler imaging demonstrates peripheral color Doppler flow without central flow. Echogenic debris centrally with lack of color flow is consistent with a cystic structure with central sloughed cells.

a neodymium:yttrium-aluminum-garnet laser is delivered using 6 to 10 W of power using a continuous mode (**Fig. 8**). Color Doppler flow can be used to track the effect of the laser energy in real time. As the laser is applied over a 5- to 20-second span, the coagulative effect is visible expanding from a few millimeters to 1.5 cm from the tip of the fiber. Using this technique, the lesion can be coagulated by region or vessel. Direct results are visible as the Doppler flow detected decreases and echogenicity of the surrounding tissue increases. Care must be taken to avoid any significant heating of the overlying skin or mucosa because bleeding and tissue loss are both possible. Great care must also be taken with higher flow lesions because air may be draw into catheters if left open and air embolus may result. Intralesional therapy can also be used as part of a multimodality approach to disease (**Fig. 9**).

Fine-Needle and Core Needle Biopsy

Fine-needle aspiration (FNA) has become a mainstay in the initial evaluation of adult lymphadenopathy. Although the pediatric malignancy spectrum makes the need for FNA less common, there are still several situations where an FNA or a core needle biopsy would be of value. Examples include enlarged parotid nodes where an

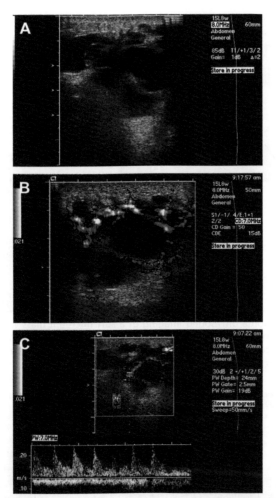

Fig. 4. (*A*) Three-year-old girl with palpable neck mass demonstrating thin-walled, multicystic masses with septae of variable thickness. Echogenic fluid may simulate solid lymph node or fluid-fluid levels may demonstrate area of recent hemorrhage into the cystic cavity. (*B*) Color power Doppler imaging demonstrates flow within the septae with (*C*) depicting an arterial waveform within septations.

excisional biopsy is difficult and any situation where direct excision is contraindicated. Although most children require the addition of sedation or anesthesia to tolerate skin penetration, ultrasound-guided biopsy offers the same advantages in children as it does in adults. Direct nodal penetration can be observed and tissue can be removed from areas throughout the node (**Fig. 10**). Needle penetration is controlled and deep structures can be preserved from needle trauma. If nodal architecture is required, core needle specimens can be taken.

Localization of Botulinum Toxin Injections for Sialorrhea and Spastic Muscular Pathology

Socially disruptive sialorrhea is a common problem encountered by children with neurologic disease. Gland removal, duct rerouting, and duct ligations are all possible

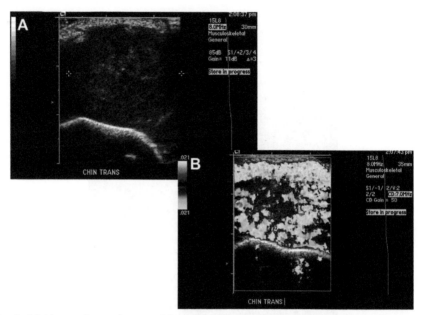

Fig. 5. (*A*) Hemangioma ultrasound imaging of a soft fluctuant mass with bluish discoloration of chin present since birth. Gray scale demonstrates slightly heterogenous hypoechogenicity with (*B*) intense diffuse color Doppler flow of the highly vascularized channels lines by endothelial cells, characteristic for hemangioma.

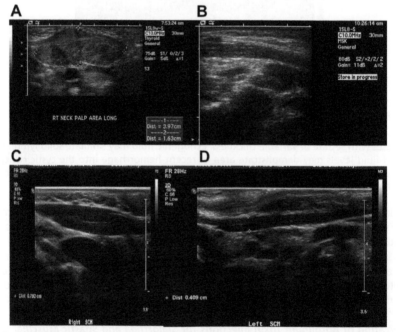

Fig. 6. Initial fibromatosis coli demonstrated by heterogenous mass entirely contained within the right SCM (*A*) with contralateral normal left SCM (*B*). Two month follow-up after physical therapy demonstrates interval improvement on the heterogenous mass (*C*) with only slight increased thickness remaining in comparison to the normal left SCM (*D*).

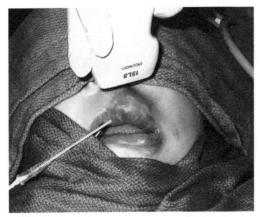

Fig. 7. A 600-μm fiber introduced via an 18-gauge angiocatheter. Tape is used to mark appropriate depth of fiber within catheter.

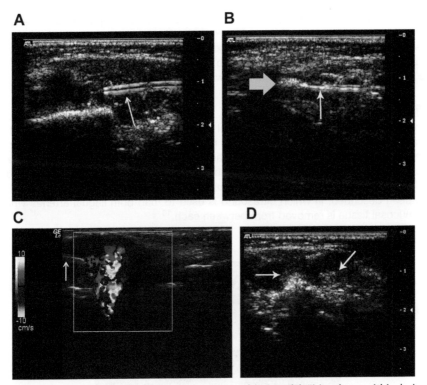

Fig. 8. (*A*) Catheter (*arrow*) visible within center of lesion. (*B*) Firing laser within lesion. Small arrow denotes 600-μm fiber protruding from catheter. Large arrow denotes increasing echogenicity of tissue as coagulation occurs. (*C*) Fiber introduced via catheter from left (*small arrow*). Color Doppler flow represents laser energy emanating from tip of fiber superiorly, artifact inferiorly. (*D*) Lesion after laser treatment. Arrows denote significant increase in echogenicity of treated areas.

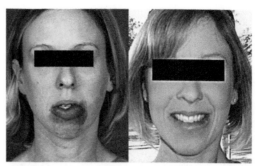

Fig. 9. Patient before and after multimodality treatment of vascular lesion. Patient underwent intralesional and pulsed dye laser treatment followed by a single debulking of the left lateral lower lip.

options but each technique is irreversible and destructive. Botox injection into the submandibular and parotid glands is a treatment that offers the patient and family a nondestructive and temporary solution. In this way, a family is able to evaluate or trial the effects of the more permanent procedures. Ultrasound is an invaluable tool for the guidance of Botox injection, which is usually done in an operating room under anesthesia. Using ultrasound localization, Botox can be directly injected into multiple areas of each gland while taking care to avoid extravasation of toxin to surrounding musculature. Identical procedures can be used to localize Botox to spastic muscle groups in the neck when treating patients for otherwise intractable disease (**Fig. 11**).

Other Potential Applications

Although many methods of airway control are familiar to pediatric otolaryngologists, ultrasound confirmation of endotracheal tube placement has been described and offers an additional potential tool.[11] Intraoperative ultrasound localization of deep neck space abscesses has been described as an adjunctive method for incision and drainage procedures.[12] Finally, minimally invasive tongue base reduction surgery has been described, in which ultrasound is used to map both lingual arteries while submucosal tissue is removed from between each.[13]

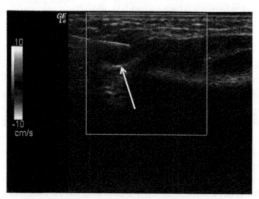

Fig. 10. Needle precisely placed within lymph node (*arrow*).

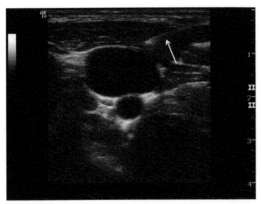

Fig. 11. Needle placed within spastic SCM muscle. Note close proximity to vasculature (*arrow*).

ULTRASOUND AS A TOOL FOR THE OTOLARYNGOLOGIST

Ultrasound, as a diagnostic modality, has been developing rapidly. High-resolution ultrasound machines have now been reduced to the size of a laptop computer. In years past, ultrasound use was largely limited to radiology departments but this is changing. Ultrasound can be easily adopted by otolaryngologists for use within the clinic and the operating room. Keys to adoption include training and close partnerships with radiology colleagues. Ultrasound seems to offer several particular advantages to the pediatric patient population. It is well tolerated and quickly adds a degree of precision to the physical examination. It can be done repeatedly as lesions evolve and treatment is performed. Finally, it is valuable for both guidance and therapeutic treatment of lesions in the operating room. With each of these benefits, it is likely that ultrasound use will continue to rapidly grow and evolve as a tool within the field of otolaryngology.

REFERENCES

1. Restrepo R, Oneto J, Lopez K, et al. Head and neck lymph nodes in children: the spectrum from normal to abnormal. Pediatr Radiol 2009;39(8):836–46.
2. Meuwly JY, Lepori D, Theumann N, et al. Multimodality imaging evaluation of the pediatric neck: techniques and spectrum of findings. Radiographics 2005;25(4):931–48.
3. Gupta P, Maddalozzo J. Preoperative sonography in presumed thyroglossal duct cysts. Arch Otolaryngol Head Neck Surg 2001;127(2):200–2.
4. Bothwell NE, Shvidler J, Cable BB. Acute rise in methicillin-resistant Staphylococcus aureus infections in a coastal community. Otolaryngol Head Neck Surg 2007;137(6):942–6.
5. Inman JC, Rowe M, Ghostine M, et al. Pediatric neck abscesses: changing organisms and empiric therapies. Laryngoscope 2008;118(12):2111–4.
6. Maddalozzo J, Goldenberg JD. Pseudotumor of infancy—the role of ultrasonography. Ear Nose Throat J 1996;75(4):248–54.
7. Friedman EM. Role of ultrasound in the assessment of vocal cord function in infants and children. Ann Otol Rhinol Laryngol 1997;106(3):199–209.
8. Bryson PC, Leight WD, Zdanski CJ, et al. High-resolution ultrasound in the evaluation of pediatric recurrent respiratory papillomatosis. Arch Otolaryngol Head Neck Surg 2009;135(3):250–3.

9. Discolo CM, Byrd MC, Bates T, et al. Ultrasonic detection of middle ear effusion: a preliminary study. Arch Otolaryngol Head Neck Surg 2004;130(12):1407–10.

10. Brietzke S, Therberge D, Mair E. Nd:YAG interstitial laser therapy for pediatric arteriovenous malformations. Operat Tech Otolaryngol Head Neck Surg 2001; 12(4):239–44.

11. Galicinao J, Bush AJ, Godambe SA. Use of bedside ultrasonography for endotracheal tube placement in pediatric patients: a feasibility study. Pediatrics 2007; 120(6):1297–303.

12. Duque CS, Guerra L, Roy S. Use of intraoperative ultrasound for localizing difficult parapharyngeal space abscesses in children. Int J Pediatr Otorhinolaryngol 2007;71(3):375–8.

13. Maturo SC, Mair EA. Submucosal minimally invasive lingual excision: an effective, novel surgery for pediatric tongue base reduction. Ann Otol Rhinol Laryngol 2006;115(8):624–30.

Emerging Technology in Head and Neck Ultrasonography

Michael R. Holtel, MD[a,b,*]

KEYWORDS
- Ultrasound technology • Microbubbles
- Ultrasound hemostasis • Head and neck ultrasound
- Elastography

ULTRASOUND: CURRENT AND FUTURE USE

Ultrasonography of the head and neck is currently a cost-effective imaging tool allowing assessment beyond the clinician's physical examination. Ultrasonography is uniquely portable when compared with other imaging modalities, making it ideal for use in the clinical setting. It provides the clinician immediate feedback, allowing the provider to make accurate assessments in a timely manner. Ultrasonography does not carry the risk of irradiation and has been the tool of choice for diagnostic and therapeutic interventions, such as fine-needle aspiration and line placement.

Ultrasound technology has distinct advantages in these areas, with continued advances and new technology likely to emerge. To allow increased ease of use in the clinical settling, palm-sized ultrasound machines are being produced, which are likely to be miniaturized even further. The ability to palpate with the ultrasound probe provides unique information on a lesion's compressibility or stiffness not available with computerized tomography (CT) and magnetic resonance imaging (MRI). This "objective" palpation is proving useful in determining whether a lesion is benign or malignant. Although attempts to use ultrasonography for therapeutic intervention in the head and neck date back to its use in Ménière disease in 1960,[1] it is in therapeutic intervention that future applications show the most promise. Two promising therapeutic ultrasound interventions are the use of (1) drug-containing *microbubbles* that, using ultrasound, can release an antitumor agent, deliver gene therapy, or release other therapeutic

The views expressed are those of the author and do not represent the views of the US Army, US military, Sharp Rees Stealy Medical Group or the University of Hawaii.

[a] Telemedicine Research Institute, University of Hawaii, 651 Ilalo Street, Honolulu, HI 96813, USA

[b] Telemedicine and Advanced Technology Research Center of the United States Army Medical Readiness and Materiel Command, MCMR-TT (TATRC) Building 1054 Patchel Street, Ft Detrick, MD 21702-5012, USA

* Sharp Rees Stealy Medical Group, 10670 Wexford Street, San Diego, CA 92131.

E-mail address: mholtel@gmail.com

substances at the target tissue and (2) focused ultrasound to coagulate bleeding vessels or destroy inaccessible tumors.

Discussions on emerging technology in ultrasonography in this article are limited to those in which there is clinical evidence to support the benefit, although in some cases that evidence is not specific to the head and neck.

MACHINE SIZE

Laptop ultrasound systems are increasingly common. Several manufacturers are introducing palm-sized ultrasound machines, including the Acuson P10 (Siemens Medical Solutions Inc, Malvern, PA, USA) introduced in 2007, the Signos (Signotics Inc, Palo Alto, CA, USA) introduced in 2009, and the Vscan (GE Healthcare, Piscataway, NJ, USA) in 2010. Although the palm-sized machines are currently designed for vascular access, bladder examination, and trauma settings, it is likely that they will eventually be improved to provide the image quality necessary for use in head and neck examination (**Fig. 1**).

PALPATION WITH ELASTOGRAPHY

Ultrasound examiners have long used palpation of masses with the ultrasound probe as an adjunct to their visual examination. Ultrasound elastography provides a more objective measurement of stiffness or, in more precise physics terms, strain. Changes in returning echoes are measured at the transducer before being converted to B-mode

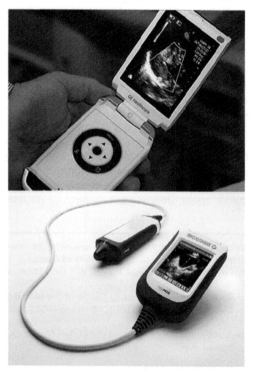

Fig. 1. Palm-sized ultrasound machines. (*Courtesy of* Signotics Inc, USA [Web site: superdupertech.com/2009/05]; with permission.)

ultrasound before and after compression with the ultrasound transducer. The difference is depicted on an elastogram as lighter for less dense and darker for more dense tissue or masses (**Figs. 2** and **3**). Since its approval by US Food and Drug Administration in 2006, ultrasound elastography has been used to discriminate between malignant and benign breast masses based on its objective measure of the stiffness of those masses. There is initial evidence that ultrasound elastography may be useful in differentiating between benign and malignant thyroid nodules. Scoring tissue stiffness on ultrasound elastography from 1 (low stiffness) to 6 (high stiffness), Hong and colleagues[2] in 2009 demonstrated in 90 consecutive surgical patients that 86 of 96 benign thyroid nodules (90%) had a score of 1 to 3, whereas 43 of 49 malignant thyroid nodules (88%) had a score of 4 to 6. Similarly, Rago and colleagues[3] in 2007 used a scoring from 1 to 5 based on elastography in 92 consecutive patients undergoing thyroidectomy for compressive symptoms or suspicion of malignancy. Low stiffness scores of 1 and 2 were found in 49 cases, all benign thyroid nodules; scores of 3, in 13 cases, one malignant and 12 benign thyroid lesions; and high stiffness scores of 4 and 5, in 30 cases, all carcinomas. Sensitivity in these 2 studies ranged from 88% to 90% and specificity, from 90% to 100%. Asteria and colleagues[4] in 2008 in a third study of 67 patients with 86 thyroid nodules used stiffness scores of 1 through 4 and found slightly higher specificity for malignancy of 94%, but a decreased sensitivity of 81%. There remains some doubt over interobserver reliability of ultrasound elastography for the thyroid nodule.

REPLACING PALPATION WITH SOUND USING SONOELASTOGRAPHY AND ACOUSTIC RADIATION FORCE IMAGING

In place of manual palpation (displacement) with the transducer, sonoelastography uses Doppler ultrasound to detect movement in a neck mass created by an external vibration. Lyshchik and colleagues[5] in 2007 examined 141 cervical lymph nodes in 43 patients with suspected hypopharyngeal or thyroid cancer using ultrasound

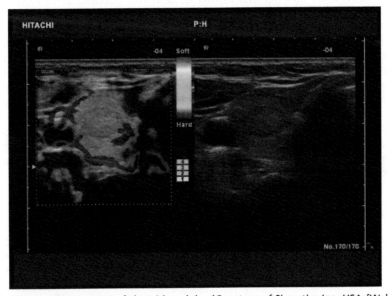

Fig. 2. Elastography images of thyroid nodule. (*Courtesy of* Signotics Inc, USA [Web site: superdupertech.com/2009/05]; with permission.)

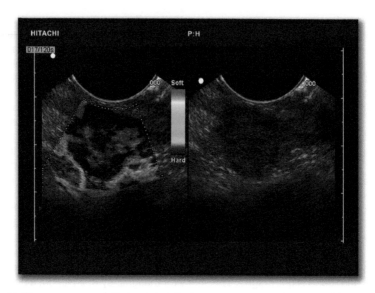

Fig. 3. Malignant upper mediastinal lymph node in esophageal carcinoma. (*Courtesy of Hitachi Medical Systems, Europe* [Web site: http://www.hitachi-medical-systems.eu/products-and-services/ct.html]; with permission.)

sonoelastography. Stiffness or strain of the lymph node and surrounding muscle was measured. When the ratio of muscle/lymph node strain was greater than 1.5, they found a 98% specificity, 85% sensitivity, and 92% overall accuracy of identifying metastatic lymph nodes. Dighe and colleagues[6] used compression generated by the carotid artery on thyroid masses along with Doppler ultrasound to determine stiffness or strain in 53 patients with thyroid lesions. This obviated a vibration source external to the neck, and they were able to distinguish 10 papillary carcinomas from 43 other thyroid lesions based on the stiffness.

Acoustic radiation force impulse (AFRI) imaging uses short-duration ultrasound pulses (0.03 to 0.4 ms) to create tissue movement/displacement and recovery, which is recorded with ultrasound correlation or Doppler ultrasound. There are no clinical studies of the head and neck, but AFRI has been used to better identify isoechoic lesions within the liver, stiffness of the heart myocardium, solid versus cystic lesions in the pancreas, and luminal intestinal lesions. Certainly, there is a potential value within the head and neck. One of the early concerns of ARFI is heat produced at the transducer and tissue being examined. Advances in AFRI beam sequencing and parallel imaging have shortened acquisition time and reduced transducer heating significantly, reducing this concern.[7]

COMBINING LIGHT AND SOUND IN PHOTOACOUSTIC IMAGING

Photoacoustic imaging (PAI) was designed to detect tissue vascularity more precisely. In PAI, a nonionizing laser targets human chromophores, such as hemoglobin and melanin, heating the tissue and causing expansion then contraction, which, in turn, gives off detectable ultrasonic waves. These ultrasonic waves are collected by an ultrasound transducer and produce an ultrasound image. In a limited study of 3 patients with port-wine stains, Kolkman[8] in 2008 demonstrated advantages in more precisely determining vascular layer and lesion depths of these vascular lesions. Nanoparticles, such as gold nanorods, shells, and cages, are particularly sensitive to light stimulation. They are being used to increase sensitivity of PAI,[9] but there are no clinical studies specific to the head and neck as yet.

CONTRAST-ENHANCING ULTRASOUND WITH MICROBUBBLES

Doppler imaging does not show capillary blood flow. Using 3- to 5-micron air bubbles or microbubbles injected intravenously to reflect the ultrasound waves provides increased vascular detail not available with Doppler imaging. Differences in microcirculation have been shown to be useful in differentiating metastatic from benign cervical lymph nodes (Zenk, 2007).[10] Examples of current commercially available microbubble contrast agents used within the head and neck include Sonovue and Sonazoid. Sonovue consists of 2.5-micron sulfur hexafluoride microbubbles stabilized with phospholipids and lasting in suspension up to 6 hours. It is commonly used in echocardiography but has also been used in imaging micrometastases in cervical lymph nodes. Sonazoid consists of perfluorocarbon with a surfactant stabilizing shell, which, when injected intravascularly, is taken up by the macrophages of the reticuloendothelial system. In the animal model, it has been injected at the tumor site to detect sentinel lymph node metastasis with 90% sensitivity as compared with 81% sensitivity in lymphoscintigraphy.[11] Both canine and porcine animal studies have found contrast-enhanced ultrasound effective in sentinel lymph node biopsy within the head and neck.[12,13] Without contrast, high-resolution ultrasound detected only 45.8% of positive neck sentinel lymph nodes in a recent large clinical melanoma study.[14]

Beyond enhancing ultrasonic images, microbubbles can have target ligands on their surface so that they are concentrated in a specific anatomic area of interest and may contain drugs for targeted delivery or even DNA plasmids to be released for gene therapy. Microbubbles can be used for thrombolysis by enhancing enzymatic thrombolytic action. Clinical trials are currently under way using mechanical pressure waves generated by transcranial ultrasound to break up clots (sonothrombolysis) and increase penetration of the thrombolytic enzyme recombinant tissue plasminogen activator (tPA).[15] Tsivgoulis and colleagues[16] performed a meta-analysis on the safety and efficacy of sonothrombolysis and found that it was not associated with any increased risk of "rebleed" and that there was a higher recanalization rate with the addition of microbubbles than with tPA alone. Ultrasound-stimulated motion of microbubbles enhances permeability across cell membranes, and endothelium provides better drug delivery which is likely to prove useful in the future for other drugs.[17]

HIGH-INTENSITY FOCUSED ULTRASOUND SURGERY

High-intensity focused ultrasound (HIFU) surgery is being developed for clinical use in hepatic, renal, prostate, and intracranial surgery, but the head and neck is certainly a possible future application as strategies to limit collateral damage in adjacent tissue are refined. HIFU creates tissue destruction through heating up the tissue and creating a coagulation necrosis with a focal acoustic lens at very low frequencies (1 to 1.5 MHz). Because of the focused nature of the ultrasound beam, the heat gradient for surrounding tissues drops off rapidly, but there can be difficulty with often cigar-shaped focal zones and damage to nearby tissue. This is of particular concern in the head and neck, because of the close proximity of critical structures. Further increasing the intensity of the HIFU can cause cavitations within the cells resulting in cell destruction. Histotripsy is an ultrasound-based strategy in the renal model that uses high-frequency ultrasound to produce cavitations with minimal heat production, thereby minimizing the risk of thermal damage to adjacent tissue.[18] In an attempt to better monitor the thermal damage to surrounding brain tissue, Jolesz and colleagues[19] have successfully used 1.5-tesla MRI that can detect changes of 3° in conjunction with HIFU applied intracranially. HIFU has also been used to occlude renal arteries in an animal model[20] and has potential usefulness in hemostasis and vessel occlusion.

THREE-DIMENSIONAL ULTRASOUND IMAGING WITHIN THE HEAD AND NECK

With an intrauterine assessment of facial abnormalities, Tonni and colleagues[21] in 2005 found three-dimensional (3D) ultrasound imaging superior to 2D in the intra-uterine fetal detection of cleft lip and palate defects and advocate its routine use for screening in the second trimester of pregnancy. Imaging of the head and neck commonly uses 3D reconstructions in computed tomography (CT) and MRI for vascular tumors, reconstruction after facial trauma, and complex masses. Both 3- and 4D (using time or video as the fourth dimension) ultrasound images are poten-tially useful for head and neck tumor assessment and detection. In a very limited study, Carraro and colleagues[22] used 3D ultrasound images enhanced with contrast microbubbles to characterize the vasculature and volume of 4 benign and 4 malignant thyroid nodules, demonstrating a higher internal vasculature in the malignant (52.3% ± 15.7%) than the benign (14.3% ± 5.3%). Zhou and colleagues[23] calculated a tumor vascularity index using a combination of 2D and 3D Doppler ultrasound of 87 patients with laryngeal carcinoma to predict cervical lymph node metastases and found a 98% specificity and 95% sensitivity.

TECHNIQUES TO SUPPRESS IMAGE ARTIFACT

Spatial compounding (SonoCT; Philips Healthcare, Andover, MA, USA) scans a lesion at different angles in real time to minimize artifact. It can "compound" up to 9 images to eliminate scatter artifact and give a more accurate image. Harmonic imaging (THI) uses integer multiples of the tissues' fundamental frequency based on the principle that these harmonic integers or overtones increase initially with increasing depth of tissue. Their increase in strength with depth lessens the effect of image artifact. Manipulations of the harmonics using second harmonics and broadband inversion techniques (Ensemble THI) further reduce image artifact. Using the fundamental frequency of microbubbles along with THI has an synergistic effect on image quality and has been called contrast harmonic imaging. Techniques to improve image quality are likely to be developed in the future.[24]

REAL-TIME IMAGE-GUIDED SURGERY

Helbig and colleagues[25] have developed a prototype for use in real-time image-guided navigational surgery, which may prove useful in soft-tissue surgery of the neck. This would provide the ability to surgically navigate from the current anatomic relationships, not relying on the preoperative relationships as in currently used CT and MRI navigational systems. There is also the potential to combine CT and ultra-sound in image-guided navigational surgery for added information, because CT and MRI are currently combined in specific surgical cases.

INCREASING USE OF ULTRASOUND

With the increasing popularity of ultrasonography performed by the clinician directly caring for the patient, there will be a demand for smaller machines with better imaging. Future modifications to improve image quality similar to Harmonic imaging and "compounding images" to reduce artifact will only accelerate ultrasound's clinical use. Use of 3D and 4D ultrasound will likely expand, but currently is limited to complex images. Supplementing the physical exam in real-time to include more information on benign versus malignant lesions, is where current emerging technology in ultrasound is likely to make a significant impact. Using objective palpation of tumor or lymph node stiffness coupled with additional tissue vascular detail using microbubbles would undoubtedly enhance the ability to distinguish benign from malignant. Success in the animal model point to the potential use of microbubbles and ultrasound in sentinel lymph node biopsy. Combining imaging modalities such as MRI with Ultrasound and Laser stimulation to provide better ultrasound imaging (Photoacoustic imaging) is providing better information than these entities used alone.

Dramatic advancement is likely in the realm of therapeutic intervention. Although the promise of coagulating bleeders with HIFU has great appeal, this area has been researched for some time and has yet to be perfected. The most impressive possibilities are in the area of targeted microbubble delivery of drugs and DNA plasmids. The ability to attach ligands to microbubbles and have relatively precise delivery of therapeutic medical interventions coupled with ultrasound's ability to increase cell penetration holds great promise for the therapeutic use of ultrasound.

REFERENCES

1. James JA, Dalton GA, Bullen MA, et al. The ultrasonic treatment of Meniere's disease. J Laryngol Otol 1960;74:730–57.
2. Hong Y, Liu X, Li Z, et al. Real-time ultrasound elastography in the differential diagnosis of benign and malignant thyroid nodules. J Ultrasound Med 2009; 28(7):861–7.
3. Rago T, Santini F, Scutari M, et al. Elastography: new developments in ultrasound for predicting malignancy in thyroid nodules. J Clin Endocrinol Metab 2007;92(8): 2917–22.
4. Asteria C, Giovanardi A, Pizzocaro A, et al. US-elastography in the differential diagnosis of benign and malignant thyroid nodules. Thyroid 2008;18(5): 523–31.
5. Lyshchik A, Higashi T, Asato R, et al. Cervical lymph node metastases: diagnosis at sonoelastography–initial experience. Radiology 2007;243(1):258–67.
6. Dighe M, Bae U, Richardson ML, et al. Differential diagnosis of thyroid nodules with US elastography using carotid artery pulsation. Radiology 2008;248(2): 662–9.
7. Hsu SJ, Bouchard RR, Dumont DM, et al. Novel acoustic radiation force impulse imaging methods for visualization of rapidly moving tissue. Ultrason Imaging 2009;31(3):183–200.
8. Kolkman RG, Mulder MJ, Glade CP, et al. Photoacoustic imaging of port-wine stains. Lasers Surg Med 2008;40(3):178–82.
9. Yang X, Stein EW, Ashkenazi S, et al. Nanoparticles for photoacoustic imaging. Wiley Interdiscip Rev Nanomed Nanobiotechnol 2009;1(4):360–8.
10. Zenk J, Bozzato A, Hornung J, et al. Neck lymph nodes: prediction by computer-assisted contrast medium analysis? Ultrasound Med Biol 2007;33:246–53.

11. Stramare R, Scagliori E, Mannucci M, et al. The role of contrast-enhanced gray-scale ultrasonography in the differential diagnosis of superficial lymph nodes. Ultrasound Q 2010;26(1):45–51.
12. Lurie DM, Seguin B, Schneider PD, et al. Contrast-assisted ultrasound for sentinel lymph node detection in spontaneously arising canine head and neck tumors. Invest Radiol 2006;41(4):415–21.
13. Curry JM, Bloedon E, Malloy KM, et al. Ultrasound-guided contrast-enhanced sentinel node biopsy of the head and neck in a porcine model. Otolaryngol Head Neck Surg 2007;137(5):735–41.
14. Sanki A, Uren RF, Moncrieff M, et al. Targeted high-resolution ultrasound is not an effective substitute for sentinel lymph node biopsy in patients with primary cutaneous melanoma. J Clin Oncol 2009;27(33):5614–9.
15. Rubiera M, Alexandrov AV. Sonothrombolysis in the management of acute ischemic stroke. Am J Cardiovasc Drugs 2010;10(1):5–10.
16. Tsivgoulis G, Eggers J, Ribo M, et al. Safety and efficacy of ultrasound-enhanced thrombolysis: a comprehensive review and meta-analysis of randomized and nonrandomized studies. Stroke 2010;41(2):280–7.
17. Stride EP, Coussios CC. Cavitation and contrast: the use of bubbles in ultrasound imaging and therapy. Proc Inst Mech Eng H 2010;224(2):171–91.
18. Klatte T, Marberger M. High-intensity focused ultrasound for the treatment of renal masses: current status and future potential. Curr Opin Urol 2009;19(2):188–91.
19. Jagannathan J, Sanghvi N, Crum L, et al. High-intensity focused ultrasound surgery of the brain: part 1–A historical perspective with modern applications. Neurosurgery 2009;64(2):201–10 [discussion: 210–1].
20. Rove KO, Sullivan KF, Crawford ED. High-intensity focused ultrasound: ready for primetime. Urol Clin North Am 2010;37(1):27–35 [table of contents].
21. Tonni G, Centini G, Rosignoli L. Prenatal screening for fetal face and clefting in a prospective study on low-risk population: can 3- and 4-dimensional ultrasound enhance visualization and detection rate? Oral Surg Oral Med Oral Pathol Oral Radiol Endod 2005;100(4):420–6.
22. Carraro R, Molinari F, Deandrea M, et al. Characterization of thyroid nodules by 3-D contrast-enhanced ultrasound imaging. Conf Proc IEEE Eng Med Biol Soc 2008;2008:2229–32.
23. Zhou J, Shang-Yong Z, Ruo-Chuan L, et al. Vascularity index of laryngeal cancer derived from 3-D ultrasound: a predicting factor for the in vivo assessment of cervical lymph node status. Ultrasound Med Biol 2009;35(10):1596–600.
24. Hoefer M. Ultrrasound teaching manual. 2nd edition. Theme; 2005. p.120.
25. Helbig M, Krysztoforski K, Krowick P, et al. Development of prototype for navigated real-time sonography for the head and neck region. Head Neck 2008; 30(2):215–21.

Index

Note: Page numbers of article titles are in **boldface** type.

A

Abscess(es), in children, 1257–1259
    subcutaneous, 1172, 1173
Absorbance, limitation of potential depth of penetration and, 1153
Acoustic impedance, and reflectance, 1152–1153
Acoustic radiation force imaging, and sonoelastography, for replacement of palpation
    with sound, 1269–1270
Adenomas, parathyroid, 1197–1201, 1230, 1231
    pleomorphic, 1179
Anterior triangle, 1162
Artifacts, multipath, 1158
    physics of, 1158–1159
    shadowing, 1158, 1159
Attenuation, 1158
    as source of energy loss, 1153
    of sound energy within tissues, frequency of sound and, 1154
    of sound wave, measurement of, 1153
Audible range, 1150

B

B-scale ultrasonography, 1154
    artifacts in, 1158
Botulinum toxin injections, localization of, for sialorrhea and spastic muscular
    pathology, 1261–1264, 1265
Brachial cleft, anomalies of, in children, 1256
Brachial cleft cyst, 1180, 1181

C

Calculus, obstructing, of ductal system, 1175, 1176
Carcinoma, anaplastic, of thyroid, 1220–1221
    follicular, of thyroid, 1218, 1219
    medullary, of thyroid, 1219–1220
    papillary, 1184, 1186, 1187, 1188, 1194, 1196–1197, 1217–1218, 1219
Carotid artery, anomalies of, 1191, 1192
    atherosclerosis of, 1188, 1191
Carotid triangular/muscle triangle (levels 2, 3, 4), 1164–1165
Cervical cysts, 1179–1182

Otolaryngol Clin N Am 43 (2010) 1275–1281
doi:10.1016/S0030-6665(10)00209-4
0030-6665/10/$ – see front matter © 2010 Elsevier Inc. All rights reserved.

oto.theclinics.com

Moving?

Make sure your subscription moves with you!

To notify us of your new address, find your **Clinics Account Number** (located on your mailing label above your name), and contact customer service at:

Email: journalscustomerservice-usa@elsevier.com

800-654-2452 (subscribers in the U.S. & Canada)
314-447-8871 (subscribers outside of the U.S. & Canada)

Fax number: 314-447-8029

Elsevier Health Sciences Division
Subscription Customer Service
3251 Riverport Lane
Maryland Heights, MO 63043

*To ensure uninterrupted delivery of your subscription, please notify us at least 4 weeks in advance of move.

Printed and bound by CPI Group (UK) Ltd, Croydon, CR0 4YY

03/10/2024

01040450-0016